T0187237

THE MAPS WE CARRY

Rose Cartwright is a screenwriter whose memoir, *Pure*, about her life with intrusive sexual thoughts, was adapted for Channel 4. She is a writer on the Netflix sci-fi series, *3 Body Problem*. Her writing about psychedelics, consciousness and mental health has been published in *The Face*, *Vice* and the *Guardian*.

Also by Rose Cartwright

Pure

THE MAPS
WE CARRY

ROSE CARTWRIGHT

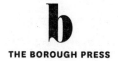

THE BOROUGH PRESS

The Borough Press
An imprint of HarperCollins*Publishers* Ltd
1 London Bridge Street
London SE1 9GF

www.harpercollins.co.uk

HarperCollins*Publishers*
Harper Ireland
Macken House,
39/40 Mayor Street Upper,
Dublin 1
D01 C9W8

First published in Great Britain by HarperCollins*Publishers* 2024
1

A catalogue record for this book is available from the British Library

HB ISBN: 978-0-00-859188-5
TPB ISBN: 978-0-00-859189-2

Typeset in Adobe Garamond Pro by Palimpsest Book Production Limited,
Falkirk, Stirlingshire

Printed and bound in the UK using 100% Renewable Electricity
at CPI Group (UK) Ltd

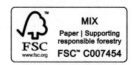

For Claire

'What we have no words for, we cannot understand. It does not fit into our view of what is real. And if we stumble upon it . . . we may be taken by surprise and frightened. On the unknown places of their maps, the ancient cartographers wrote, "here there be dragons"'.[1]

Jack Kornfield, Buddhist teacher

Intentions

This morning we sat in a circle, took a deep breath, and set our intentions. Some intended to heal, others to surrender. There were tears and respectful silences and nods of understanding.

Now we take the magic mushrooms and everything goes dark. For the next two hours I watch my identity slide like guts. There is nothing with any recognisable form, only an endless churn of organic textures I cannot identify. Nothing, including me, has ever existed, only a single emotion: primal fear. Later, I push through into a vast space of light where love has a physical materiality that I can touch and of which every cell in my body is made. Orchestral music builds as my heart is broken wide open and I weep tears of love for the people around me. One of them has regressed to infancy and rocks back and forth. Another holds their head. Another sways softly, whispering to themselves. Another sheds ecstatic tears.

I take in the scene and have a thought: 'What a bunch of assholes.'

I burst out laughing and turn away.

Someone is groaning like a child. Someone else sighs in bliss, unselfconsciously loud.

'When are these assholes going to shut up?' I say, pressing my face into the pillow, unearthing all of the laughter that's been fossilising at the back of silent classrooms and solemn churches and po-faced yoga studios, where I buried it in layers over years, along with many other miscellaneous inappropriate thoughts and feelings.

I cover my mouth and laugh through my fingers as someone to my left battles an inner demon. His wailing is genuinely irritating, insufferably irritating, and I find myself wishing that he would re-repress some of that generational pain so that I can get a moment's peace. Trying to stop the laughter only makes it worse.

What this means to me (the hypocrisy and sheer unreasonableness of slinging fatuous insults at friends during their most unguarded and transcendent moments) is unfolding with a wicked rush of revelatory energy. I see into the mechanics of the laughter and understand what I'm supposed to understand: that I can only find this funny because the love between me and these people is unquestioned, and that it is at this biting point of mutually-informing reverence and irreverence that I know I must try to write this book.

It's something I had been puzzling over (psychedelics have a mysterious ability to catalyse the solving of puzzles): how do I criticise our mental health system with the scathingness that feels necessary, while also respecting the people working within it? How do I challenge psychiatry's framing of serious distress as disease, while honouring what that framing means to people? How do I appraise the ways in which my own ignorance has perpetuated unhelpful stories about mental health, while also showing myself compassion? How do I construct as much as I deconstruct? Offer hope as much as I call bullshit? I can only do this if there's a mutual understanding between us from the outset that my critique comes from a place of love, and that it is my intention to write from that place.

~

We are all searching for a story, an orienting narrative that shows us our place in the world. We use the tools of storytelling to make sense of ourselves. We keep a lookout for through-lines and patterns, recurring themes and the opening and closing of chapters. Perhaps you have a sense of the person you were, the person you are, and the person you'd like to be, as well as the consistent 'you', the central character, who has made mistakes, learned lessons and evolved along the way.

Within our stories, we use metaphor to give ourselves a landscape through which to unfold: plateaus, peaks, forks in the road, deserts, new horizons and rocky patches. Some people are able to navigate their inner landscape with a sense of exploration. Some of us are easily lost; our world has a strange incoherency, familiar and unfamiliar at once, homely in its unhomeliness. The maps we carry seem to sabotage us with wrong turns, and the ways out seem impossibly steep. When we're stuck like this, disruption can be helpful.

Altered states of consciousness have been used by humans for tens of thousands of years to disrupt our habitual ways of seeing things.[1] They can happen spontaneously and unbidden, or they can be induced and cultivated, alone or in group settings, by activities like sleep deprivation, extreme heat and cold, meditation, lucid dreaming, sex, breathwork, chanting, drumming, dancing, fasting, contemplation, and psychedelic drugs.[2] They are sometimes called mystical experiences, non-ordinary states of consciousness or transpersonal states of consciousness.

Psychologist Abraham Maslow studied what he called 'peak experiences' in depth, noting reports of bliss and euphoria, sensations of warmth and vibration, a blurred sense of time and space and expansive connectedness with others and the universe.[3] Writer Malidoma Somé described ecstatic trances in his accounts of initiation ceremonies in Burkina Faso. For his tribespeople, these trances meant voyages into other worlds and communion with spirits.[4] The accounts of nineteenth-century Indian mystics Ramakrishna and Vivekananda, with their repeated references to unity with the eternal, limitlessness and unboundedness, inspired psychoanalyst Romain Rolland to coin the phrase 'the oceanic feeling' in a letter to Sigmund Freud.[5] Using only breathwork, psychiatrist Stanislav Grof induced what he called 'holotropic' states (*holo* meaning 'wholeness' and *tropic* meaning 'moving towards'), when his research drug of choice, LSD, was outlawed in the US in 1968.[6]

'Cosmic consciousness', wrote scholar Alan Watts, 'otherwise known as mystical experience, otherwise known as *moksha, nirvana, bodhi, satori, fana-al-fana* or what you will . . . happens to people. It has happened as far back as we know. It happens all over the world, and in all cultures. We don't know very much about it . . . But it unquestionably happens, and most people keep their mouths shut about it when it does.'[7]

In this book, I use altered states of consciousness to disrupt two stuck stories: the mental illness paradigm, and my trauma, which are so interrelated as to be one and the same story.

According to the dominant story of mental suffering, which I grew up with and promoted for years in my mental health advocacy, the main causes of persistent, intense distress are organic problems in our brains, problems that can be categorised like diseases and treated like them. Because this story offers reassurance and surface-level answers, and because it serves the psychiatric industry well, it's become pervasive, calcified, and resistant to interrogation. Trauma is also calcification. It similarly freezes a story about reality in time and is just as reluctant to loosen its grip. Altered states of consciousness can be good tools for softening the sclerosis of both.

When we take mind-altering drugs or do mind-altering activities, leaving behind our predictable patterns and entering more unpredictable and dream-like territory; when, to borrow language from anthropologist Gregory Bateson, our everyday prosaic consciousness stands down and we enter the poetic consciousness of an altered state,[8] rigid beliefs about the world can become more flexible, and new ways of thinking about problems can arise.

We desperately need new ways of thinking about problems in the face of our mental health crisis. The UK's Office of National Statistics reports that millions of British people are often or always lonely.[9] According to the World Health Organization (WHO), a fifth of the world's children have a mental health condition, and someone dies by suicide every forty seconds. [10] It shouldn't surprise us that the suicide rate in the UK's most deprived areas is almost double the rate of that in the most affluent.[11] In this book, I come to the conclusion that treating misery as a primarily medical problem is part of the reason why so many people are miserable. Whether or not you agree with that, we can probably all agree that something about the way we are approaching mental health isn't working, and that radical change is desperately needed.

The Maps We Carry is told through essays, articles, interviews and extracts from my journals. It unfolds over six years, 2017–23, during which time I underwent two transformations moving in lockstep: an intellectual transformation, from seeing my problems as self-annihilating symptoms of disease to self-protective strategies of survival; and an emotional transformation: from feeling suicidal to feeling fulfilled.

Altered states of consciousness (reached in various ways but most powerfully through meditation, ecstasy and magic mushrooms) were catalysts, not cures, and cannot be understood in isolation from my life, where supportive loved ones, financial privilege, professional satisfaction, and a skilled psychotherapist all contributed inextricably. While I would welcome the legalisation of psychedelics, I'm concerned about these drugs being plugged into psychiatry as it stands, where brain is decontextualised from body, present from past, science from traditional knowledge, individual story from social story. This book will look at the ways disadvantaged groups suffer when context is overlooked. Spoiler alert: psychedelics don't solve systemic social problems.

Three scenes are fictionalised versions of conversations that happened either in real life or in my imagination. I've written them in screenplay format to distinguish them from the rest of the book, which is factual. I've occasionally changed names and identifying details to protect people's privacy.

I work as a writer in TV, film and books. My first memoir, *Pure*, in which I wrote about my experience of intrusive sexual and violent thoughts as a symptom of obsessive compulsive disorder, came out in 2015 and boosted my profile as a mental health advocate. Through my advocacy, I promoted a set of ideas which I thought to be true: that mental illnesses are illnesses like any other; that mental illnesses can be scientifically categorised into diagnoses; that one in four people in the world has a mental illness. When I started to have these ideas challenged, I was resistant at first. I wrote this book to try to write myself out of my disillusionment; to find a new positioning system, a new way to orientate to suffering that didn't involve 'illness'. Without a coherent cultural story about what my suffering meant, I used what I had closest to me – my knowledge of story – to try to structure a healing experience.

~

The topic of mental health is inscrutable and impossibly complex, 'a beguiling mystery and brutally difficult' as a friend and mentor said to me. It's nothing less than the question of who we are and why we suffer, and any single model of understanding is bound to be reductive. The biomedical model, which tackles distress like pathology, has so far generally failed to improve people's lives, and though the trauma model (the idea that suffering is the result of exposure in the past to adversity) is more common sensical and backed by more evidence, it too can be reductive. As Maslow famously said, 'If the only tool you have is a hammer, it is tempting to treat everything as if it were a nail.'[12] Sometimes we hunt for causal agents in the past because we can't see the normalised dysfunction in the present. Sometimes the search for ways in which we've been victimised can blind us to our considerable agency. The shift away from the biomedical model to the trauma model (which is now happening culturally but hardly at the level of healthcare) is often characterised as a shifting question: from 'what's wrong with you?' to 'what happened to you?'. I broadly agree with the direction, but I'd add a couple more questions: 'what *is* happening to you?' and 'what role are you playing in perpetuating it?'.

This book is not an endorsement of psychedelics. The drugs are illegal in most places and they're not for everyone. Though they can be immensely powerful in helping us to become unstuck, the psychological risks are real and serious. Even when taken under optimal conditions, psychedelics can destabilise fragile minds and lead to long-lasting anxiety, confusion, hallucinations, and derealisation. However, harm has also come from fearmongering around the dangers of psychedelics. When used in supportive settings, psychedelics are, in the majority of cases and even when they profoundly challenge us, safe, and statistically far less harmful than alcohol, the nation's favourite drug.

How I see psychedelics will be different to how you see them. This is an inescapably subjective story, not a manual that you can follow. Mental health science makes the mistake of trying to get around people's subjectivity so that it can apparently arrive at objective conclusions. I'm of the view that any 'treatment' must embrace and work through a person's subjectivity, not iron it out as though it were an inconvenience or dismiss it as placebo. Though the focus of this book is on psychedelics and mental health, I don't primarily see these drugs as medicines. I think they're valuable as conduits to have fun, goof around, let off steam, explore the weird and the dangerous, connect with others and with nature, philosophise, grieve, find creative inspiration and mark rites of passage. Because our various shades of despair have been framed as illnesses that need treating by professionals rather than problems that need preventing through community, we've drawn an unhelpful and arbitrary line between therapy and recreation. While good psychotherapy, if you're lucky enough to access it and afford it, is an excellent conduit to healing through psychedelics, some of my most therapeutic altered states have been with friends in recreational settings: dancing, being silly and talking shit about the wider world, not lying down and talking to a therapist about my inner world.

~

One thing this book is not, is an attempt to analyse the science of nature or nurture in mental health. I have no scientific training, and the dichotomy seems moot, since nature and nurture are not separate. I have tried to do that research in private, attempted to figure out the extent to which I was predestined to develop mental health problems or whether I was a blank sheet of paper, or where I sat in between. You can do it too if you're interested, but it's easy to get tangled in the weeds. Experts don't agree on which factors contribute most to mental health problems. For every expert who expresses an opinion, there's another equally credentialled, articulate and respected expert who has a different take. For every study that is published in a respectable journal, there's a direct rebuttal published in another equally respectable journal. Every debunk is stridently debunked. Psychiatrists and critical psychiatrists are endlessly hashing it out on social media, the tone of which are often smug or snippy.

To the limited extent that I'm able to judge, the body of evidence that past and present exposures to stress are the leading determinants of common mental health problems like anxiety disorders, depression, PTSD and OCD,[13] is vast, whereas evidence that organic brain dysfunction or genetics are the leading causes of such conditions is comparatively scant. Many experts agree that with psychosis, schizophrenia and bipolar disorder, evidence for biological determinants is stronger,[14] though others assert that these experiences are also, at heart, responses to trauma.[15] It's important to note that many people who experience auditory and visual hallucinations do not think of themselves as having illnesses at all.[16] I should also make it clear that when I refer to 'mental health problems' in this book, I do not mean neurological conditions like Alzheimer's, or developmental conditions like autism.

Mental health is multifactorial, and our genes play a large role in our personalities and mental capacities. But it doesn't follow that I always had a latent potential for a brain disease called OCD. Despite the development of precise diagnostic tests in other branches of medicine, no biological tests can currently diagnose mental health problems. And while I can't be certain, in the broadest strokes I think the idea that we get chronically distressed because of problems with our brains, more than problems in the world, is unfounded.

I believe that science will play a vital role in the future of healing. But science is not the whole story, nor in my opinion, even half the story, of mental health. Exploring what makes us desperately unhappy is just as much a question for everyday people (whose knowledge and intuitions have for decades been systemically subjugated by psychiatric authority), for philosophers, anthropologists, politicians, and artists, as it is for scientists. Maybe we shouldn't expect science to explain mental health any more than we should expect it to explain love or grief. These are not things we can measure or capture or verify as real or not real, but they are profoundly true, and paradoxically, their mystery makes them more true, not less. Same goes, I would say, for mental health problems.

As I explored my internal life through altered states in this book, the precise language of science fell increasingly short. We don't have an agreed-upon definition of mind, or consciousness. Thought itself is inherently mysterious. There's no way to independently test that what I might describe as anxiety is what you describe as anxiety. I've come to see my mental health problems as a counterintuitive expression of love: of my need for love and belonging, and of the fear of losing those things. Do we need scientific authority to tell us about love? Or do we already have that knowledge deep in our bones somewhere? 'Do we need a story to tell us what is sacred?' asks mythologist Joseph Campbell, 'or do we already have the experience that matches the story?'[17] If we strip diagnostic language back to the raw experience of extreme distress – dark, heavy, lost, foggy, monstrous – we soon default to metaphor, our go-to mode, whether we notice it or not.

I owe a lot to mental health science. Without decades of work in psychedelics and trauma research, and the resulting zeitgeist, it's unlikely I would have found healing. I owe even more to the wisdom of traditional societies, whose participatory ways of living (community rituals, rhythmic movement, communion with nature, psychoactive plants, storytelling), and common-sense philosophies (strength in numbers, safety in numbers, resource-sharing, the present as a continuation of ancestry), offer more guidance than a century of psych research, the findings of which are often corroborating and repackaging knowledge that the West has forgotten, stolen or destroyed.

I have had the dubious privilege of having spent two decades immersing myself in a wide variety of mainstream psych treatments, including most of the major psychotherapies, many 'alternative' therapies and antidepressants. This bird's eye view has been helpful when interrogating a mental health system which is siloed by academic curricula, career paths, diagnostic categories, and insurance codes. Inevitably, mental health professionals tend to believe that their particular therapy, medicine or research area (the thing they've spent money and time training in; the thing for which they earn prestige) is what works best. Generally, they will be on board with a critique of the system until that critique is brought against their specialism. As we shall see, these incentives are part of what makes Western mental health care so abysmal and resistant to change.

In one sense, I don't think we're searching for answers about mental health. We know that we become unhappy when we're isolated from each other and from nature, when there's scarcity of resources, and when we are compelled into work that lacks meaning and maroons us further from the people we love. In another sense, when faced with any one individual's mental health, we ought to leave any assumed understanding at the door. I have no idea what you've been through and what your mind is like and why. You have a far more accurate map of your self than anyone else does. 'You're the expert on you', as my brilliant former psychotherapist Joyce Blake often reminded me.

This book tells the story of how, since writing *Pure*, I fundamentally changed what I think about mental health. But there are through-lines between that project and this one. Embracing uncertainty is one of them. It's a skill you can learn (meditation and psychedelics help): cultivating uncertainty about what our thoughts and feelings mean, and trying, in the spirit of most good psychotherapy, not to avoid what scares us. 'Certainty is the greatest of all illusions,' writes psychiatrist Iain McGilchrist. 'The only certainty, it seems to me, is that those who believe themselves to be certainly right are certainly wrong.'[18]

I've been consistent on another important point which I want to emphasise: mental health problems are real and devastating. How you feel is not your fault. You didn't choose this. You didn't imagine it or make it up. You are deserving of all the compassion and care and non-judgement that would be afforded to a person with any other kind of illness.

Take OCD, for example. The experience of having repetitive ego-dystonic thoughts that cause extreme distress, and engaging in compulsive rituals to neutralise them, is a very real and often debilitating phenomenon. Same goes for experiences that people call anxiety or depression or bipolar disorder or personality disorder – absolutely real.

We can question the validity of mental illness as a construct without taking any of that off the table. We can assert that our experiences are real while also interrogating the conceptualisation of such experiences as diseases with primarily biological determinants, the organisation of these experiences into discrete categories, and the assumption that such experiences are 'disordered', as opposed to in some way functional, i.e. adaptive responses to a disordered environment. It may sound counterintuitive, but it was only when I stopped framing my distress as the symptom of disease that I reached a deeper appreciation of its seriousness.

That said, I believe the medical model should remain an option for those that find it helpful, as long as it's signposted as a model, i.e. as a map of reality not reality itself, and therefore intrinsically limited. (A map of the coastline will be accurate in one sense, but it won't tell you anything about the essence of a beach. How the seaweed smells, the chalky sound of pebbles underfoot.) If seeking biomedical treatment has helped you map your problems and has led to lasting contentment, keep going and do whatever works – each person's way of making meaning of their own mind is valid.

This book is for those who've tried everything that the medical model has to offer, and still suffer.

A psychiatrist at South London and Maudsley, an NHS Trust that annually provides 40,000 people with mental health services (I've been one of those people), confided in me with a heavy heart that they're often treating people knowing they'll probably still be treating them in twenty years. I've heard this despondency echoed by dozens of other mental health professionals. Treatments that we're told are evidence-based don't seem to work that well in the long term, not because clinicians lack skills or expertise, but because they have such a limited range of tools. I'm writing this book because I think there are better tools out there, and better stories.

I'm interested in the functions that stories serve and the way we use story structures like physical structures. We gather around them, we use them as weapons and shields, we hang ideas off them, we live in them. When a story gets so big – like the story that mental distress is a symptom of disease – it becomes like a city, full of architecture so familiar we barely look at it. I felt compelled to write this book now because I believe that psychedelics are about to transform the way mental health problems are conceptualised, offering us a unique opportunity to stop, look around, and think deeply about the stories we've built. Which structures could be improved? Which are keepers? Which provide necessary shelter? Which could be modified? Which should be razed to ground?

The Maps We Carry is predicated on the possibility that below the level of conscious awareness, our mind–body systems intuitively understand story structure; that there is a part of all of us that is always seeking to unfold, like a story, and that the hallmarks of storycraft are uncoincidentally the hallmarks of healing from the fragmentation of trauma. Metaphor, imagery, narrative arcs, expansion and contraction, meaning-making, patterns of cause and effect. I will make the case that you, like all good stories, had the blueprint for wholeness written into you from the start. That when you are supported, trusted, empowered and loved, you know how to find your way to resolution; you know how to heal.

PART ONE

Preparation

Departure

'We exist in a terrifying vastness of unimaginable complexity. Narrative brings order to chaos. It is reassuring and makes us feel more in control. The universe is less frightening if we have a story.'[1]

Frank Tallis, psychologist

2017

I know something is starting when my breathing falls into an unfamiliar pattern. Breathing is happening but I am not doing it. The body is breathing itself and the 'I' has suddenly grown distant. The inbreaths stir tingles in my feet and the outbreaths send them up my legs in an electric wave. When the wave reaches the base of my spine, it surges up into my chest and head, and whooshes back down my limbs. Synaesthesia comes next. Noises are the same as sensations. I feel the sound of a bird screeching as a ripple up my spine, so strong it causes me to arch my back. Sparkling white lights fill my vision and a field of non-duality opens out, in which I am pure sensory texture. The thoughts that mediate experience disappear, leaving just experience. Sounds are sounds. Sight is sight. Touch is touch. There are no concepts of what these things are. No sense of a 'me' who is hearing or seeing. The faces of my parents appear above me, as if projected from somewhere behind me. Tears of joy stream down my face. The wave that started in my toes moves out to fill the room, taking the boundaries of my body with it, stretching out over the sugar pine forest and giant redwoods down to the ocean. The white light intensifies as the widening circles of my self expand across the ocean and roll back towards my body and through my chest, which is both the recipient and the source of boundless, cosmic love. I sink to my knees as the waves and the bright lights start to rescind over the horizon, before it all stops.

My vision desaturates and the material world of carpet, chair legs and skirting boards comes back into focus as I catch my breath. I look around and remember where I am. In a dormitory. On a ten-day meditation retreat in California. I'm 31 years old. It's a Saturday. I look at the clock and see that more than an hour and a half has passed. Strangely, as I look around, I have the feeling of having emerged from somewhere real into somewhere unreal.

'What the fuck was that?' I say out loud.

It felt like a mushroom trip. But I haven't taken any drugs, so how could that be possible? I've been sober for days. Besides, I wouldn't know what mushrooms feel like because I've never done them. Maybe I ate something at breakfast by accident? Unlikely. As my breathing slows, I take in more of my surroundings. Out the window I can just see the tops of the dry grass hills from where I'm lying, a bird of prey circling above, the ceiling fan going round and round.

Can you trip sober? Can you trip off your own chemicals? What happened in my brain just now?

I can feel my mind doing what it always does, reaching for the cognitive escape hatch, asking what something *is* to save me from feelings: the lifelong tendency at the heart of all my problems. There has to be a rational explanation for why a novice meditator would seem to trip into a transcendent reality and spend the best part of a couple of hours there. I've read that when you meditate for long periods and you're deprived of typical levels of sensory inputs, your brain can start to generate its own sensory stimulation.[2] Could it have been that?

I don't know in this moment what my distant ancestors would've known and what many traditional societies know still: that powerful altered states of consciousness can be cultivated without drugs; or that meditators can sometimes reach such intense levels of concentration that the apparatus of thought and ego can lift; or that shamans have been inducing altered states for millennia to disrupt ordinary ways of seeing. I don't know that altered states were probably a ritualistic part of life for the Native American Chumas that lived here in California five hundred years ago; or that the dung-burning Celts of Britain's Iron Age psychonauts – explorers of consciousness – too.

I don't have my phone so I can't look it up and I wouldn't know what to look up anyhow. Sober trip? Spontaneous spiritual experience? *Mystical* experience? I'm already rehearsing how I will describe this to friends and family in such a way that they don't think I've joined a cult. I'm not sure there is a way. The retreat is bad enough. If they could hear the *ohm*s and see the beards and the way the meditators walk ever so slowly, they would already assume I was lost. And I am lost, in a way: an atheist and a sceptic, drawn to spirituality but with no spiritual home, attracted to contemplative practices but turned off by their attendant woo woo. I'm loath even to bow to the Buddha as I've seen the other yogis doing this week, their hands clasped, their faces contorted. I'm cautious of what happens when we make idols of ideas, but I want to surrender myself to something. Lately I've been feeling uprooted from a deeper sense of connection with the world and longing for experiences that make me feel small. I'm trying with meditation, but when it comes to holistic wellness, there are barriers to entry for me. The grandiosity of self-styled gurus. The earnestness of their devotees. The ease with which conversations about breathing patterns and body alignment can slide towards the New Age. The self-serving claims made by so-called life coaches about their intuitive powers to transform me. Mediumship, astrology, manifestation, crystals. I have a tonal allergy to all of it. I've noticed that it's often the most obtuse-seeming person in the room who calls themselves – with a straight face and a breathy voice – an *empath*; and that the people who will unselfconsciously tell you that they're *doing the work* are often the people who, while living an eternal gap year of yoga retreats in Portugal, breathwork sessions in Chelsea and apothecary workshops in Somerset, seem to have scarcely done a day of actual work in their lives.

But my post-Enlightenment education with its steely materialism has left me ill-prepared for, and squeamish about, surprise moments of heart-bursting oneness with everything that exists. So more fool me.

Within seconds of coming round, a sequence of sexual thoughts about the people who were meditating beside me this morning closes in on my mind. It happens in slow motion, like the falling of a curtain. The hairs stand up on my arm as my body realises what this means before I do, then it hits my conscious mind and I curl into a ball and start sobbing. To understand why, we need to leave me here on the sun-dappled floor and

take

a

step

back.

2002

My thoughts were not like most people's thoughts. Everyone has bad ones sometimes, but mine were something else. When I was 15 years old, horrifying thoughts about child abuse started to intrude into every minute of every day, bringing with them an ambient dread that never lifted and often broke out into panic. It was the year that two 10-year-old schoolgirls were abducted and murdered in Soham, Cambridgeshire. Their pictures were in every newspaper and across every news bulletin when you turned on the TV. I was a kid myself, I didn't really understand what had happened to them, but I knew it was something horrendous, the worst possible thing. What if in the past I'd done the worst possible thing without realising? Or was capable of doing it in future? The fact I'd even asked myself that question became concrete proof to me that my thoughts represented a true threat. By 18, I was bulimic and self-harming; by 21, I was suicidal.

While this core mechanism (having a deeply distressing thought and assuming that its presence confirmed my capacity to act it out) remained, the themes changed over the years. Other preoccupations included intrusive abusive language, fears about the structural integrity of buildings, excessive doubts about my sexuality, intrusive mental images of my bones breaking as I walked, and a conviction that my face and body were physically monstrous. Utmost hypervigilance was essential in this world of cosmic fear, where every impulse could be acted upon, every ceiling could crash, every thought could be true.

Society told me a story about my suffering. It said I had a mental illness, an illness like any other, that anyone could develop and that could be treated as a physical disease. People said there was something faulty about the way my brain worked, a chemical imbalance or some overactive neural circuitry, and that this was the root cause of my problem. It said my behaviours and thoughts were the symptoms of this illness and that they weren't 'me', any more than someone's flu is them. I wasn't to blame; I was just mentally ill with a plague that served no purpose but to torment me. For centuries, the priest had been the person you went to when you were desperately unhappy, but now that science had apparently proven that unhappiness was caused by organic problems inside the brain, you had to go and see the doctor.

I don't remember the first time I heard about mental illness because it was a fact of the universe, embedded into the way things worked, like gravity. And because I'd been searching for a story, I held on to it tight. When you're confused and scared, official-sounding terms like *generalised anxiety disorder* and *depression* (the first two diagnoses I'd received having described my distressing thoughts to doctors), and existing frameworks like *assessment, treatment* and *medication*, feel like a life raft in the fog – the only thing for miles with any structure. So I grew up as someone with mental illness. I incorporated the language of medicine into my understanding of my life, to describe cycles of relapses and recoveries. The story was hopeful, because if different diseases responded to different treatments, modern medicine could treat my unhappiness.

When I was in my early twenties, while my skin was healing my self-harm cuts into scars, I googled the phrase 'intrusive thoughts', and discovered that I wasn't the only person in the world who thought such terrible things, and that the thoughts were the symptoms of an illness called OCD. Alone in my room at university, I lay on the carpet and cried with relief.

I took this new knowledge to a doctor and received a formal diagnosis of that condition. The process was so neat and so drenched in good intentions – OCD seemed to be such a fitting explanation – I didn't notice that that it had not been based on anything scientific. I would come to understand years later that my diagnosis was a co-created story, an arrived-upon subjectivity between a desperate patient and a well-meaning doctor: a patient incentivised by the search for a decisive end to pain; a doctor incentivised, perhaps, by the authority of their profession. Genuinely and effortlessly, we co-wrote a script: a mutual understanding that my previous diagnoses had clearly been misdiagnoses, but that this was finally the right one. Through some kind of interpersonal alchemy, we agreed on a past, present and intended future, and enshrined the story in paperwork as fact, where it became codified according to diagnostic manuals that had been written long ago and far away and that told a much bigger story about the medicalisation of suffering that I didn't yet understand.

2013

In ways I didn't realise, my diagnosis was leading me down a narrow path. I found a specialist OCD clinic that offered cognitive behavioural therapy. CBT says that if you change your thinking and your behaviour, your feelings will follow, and that if you expose yourself regularly enough to ideas that make you anxious, you will habituate to the fear and cease to be afraid. I believed in the formula (it was the only one I had), and the therapy seemed to work for a while.

Age 27, having kept my OCD a secret from everyone in my life for more than a decade, I wrote an article about it for a newspaper that was shared all over the world. Within days, hundreds of thousands of people had read about my battle with this devastating disease, which the World Health Organization ranked as one of the top ten most disabling illnesses of any kind.[3] The message in the article was unambiguous: you have an illness and it can be treated just like other illnesses.

The problem was, I'd made a mistake, the same mistake made by so many studies into the efficacy of mental health treatments: ignoring context that doesn't seem relevant but may be highly influential. After months of intensive exposure therapy, I'd become somewhat numbed to the content of my thoughts; had interpreted that numbness as getting better, and had chalked up the change in my mental state to the success of the therapeutic technique. All the while underestimating the role of the things that, looking back, I see were truly helping: my relationship with the therapist, my sense of control in doing something proactive, and the fact that, in my mid-twenties, I was already writing the notes that would become *Pure*. When the therapy ended, and my relational tie to my therapist was cut, and I was no longer collaborating with a trusted confidante every week (as we'll see, separation is my kryptonite), I felt the darkness close in again.

2016

Nesting did something strange to me. We'd met in our mid-twenties and planned to share a life together, but when we decided to buy a flat, the next milestone, I started to feel less solid. My foundations started to sink.

Every day, I was seeing flashing images of my ankles breaking as I walked, and of floors collapsing as I crossed them. Everything felt unsure again. The structural integrity of my self could not be trusted, especially not during any moment that was supposed to be meaningful or intimate. I'd had physical and emotional closeness undermined so many times by intrusive thoughts that a sweet nothing, handhold or kiss on the lips had become coupled with an expectation that I was about to have an unsettling thought. The feared thought would then inevitably come, and my resulting detachment would become evidence that I wanted what was in my head, not what was right in front of me. I knew that I could never get married because the moment I had to say 'I do', an intrusive thought would undermine the certainty I'd need to declare such a thing. It sounds bonkers and maddening, and it was. When flat-hunting, I refused to look at buildings that were taller than they were wide, in case they fell over in the wind. We laughed about it, but I was deadly serious. I knew the idea was irrational, but I felt the threat was real.

When we settled on a flat and began the long mortgage process, I started to pick fights, growing sullen and angry and jealous. Some days I went into total shutdown and wouldn't look at him. I knew that my behaviour was unjustified, but I felt that it was righteous, and in the gap between the knowing and the feeling, shame grew like weeds. If you'd stood on one side of that gap and shouted your rationalisations across it at the top of your voice, no one on the other side would've heard. I tried every day.

This was not how the story was supposed to go. When you've crawled through a river of shit and come out clean on the other side, you're not ever, according to the rules of good storytelling, supposed to crawl back into the pipe. As my book got picked up and my profile grew, invitations from magazines and podcasts rolled in. I received hundreds of messages of gratitude from the public, telling me how my book had inspired them to follow in my footsteps and seek the same treatments. I felt like a fraud.

'We should beware of the special price we have to pay,' writes philosopher Alain de Botton in *On Mental Illness*, 'when we have allowed ourselves to declare the battle over, when we have announced to ourselves and to friends that we are well again – and then recognise that we have actually been hasty and naive and need to return to the front once more. It can feel especially bitter to have to crouch low again when we felt we now had the right to stand tall.'[4]

If you do ever have to crouch low again and crawl back into the shitpipe, usually you do it quietly, but Channel 4 had already given the TV adaptation of *Pure* the greenlight, meaning my redemption story was already on the way to being broadcast to millions of people.

As the move-in date approached, and I watched my hands packing our belongings into separate boxes, I discovered, like I'd heard it on the radio about someone else's life, that a part of me had already decided to destroy everything that we'd built. I invented grievances to justify my leaving and punished him for emotions I didn't recognise as my own. But really, it was over nothing. It's always the nothing that's the most disturbing: the workings that aren't shown, the boardroom table in your own heart that you don't have a seat at. I'd love to have known what was going on in there. I hope they at least had croissants.

After I left, I tumbled through a series of reinvention

clichés: I cut my hair, I bought a new fragrance, I fell in love with a couple of gorgeous but disastrous men, I booked myself onto a ten-day silent meditation retreat. I managed to convince myself that my loneliness was me-time, that my directionlessness was freedom. But staying in friends' houses didn't feel like it used to. The spare room in people's lives was being filled with weddings and babies, so I moved into a flat share in east London. I unpacked the bits from my old life into my new. I hung my clothes in the wardrobe by colour. I found sunny spots on windowsills for the plants and fussed over the placement of cushions. When that was done, I curled up on the floor and cried for the part of me that could not be unpacked or *turned to face the light.*

2017

The Californian sun has moved round and is warming my skin through the dormitory window. I wipe the tears from my face with my T-shirt. They say about pilgrimages that it's not until you arrive and put down your bags that you realise the weight you've carried all the way. Now I realise.

This altered state of consciousness, this sober trip, or mystical experience, or whatever the fuck just happened, it doesn't matter what I call it. What matters, what's just dawned on me, is that for the ninety minutes just gone, I didn't have a single thought, intrusive or otherwise. It was the first time in fifteen years of treatment for mental illness that I've been fully liberated from harrowing thoughts, from that life, and from thought itself. There had been images and words, but they were a picture show happening outside of me, detached from me. There had been no internal voice silently remarking that my breathing had changed or that I was seeing lights; only the direct experience of the breathing and the seeing, unmediated by concepts, unmediated by 'me', by self, and all the reflexive ideas that the self lugs around.

I don't know if you can imagine thoughtlessness. Actually, I know you can't, since imagination itself is thought. But if, like most people, your mind is chattering away almost all of the time with unhelpful repetitive thought-loops, then you can perhaps imagine how relieved you'd be if that thinking briefly stopped and you got the chance to look at reality without referring back to your thoughts of what reality is. Then perhaps you can also imagine the deflation of going back to business as usual.

I hear the bell from the main hall announcing the end of a meditation session. I stand and splash my face with cold water. People will be back in the dorm soon; I've got to try to shake off this confusion.

I'd always been told that my intrusive thoughts were point-less symptoms, but how can the symptoms of illness spontaneously disappear and then return? There was some-thing in that moment of witnessing my thoughts lift, almost like a physical barrier – a barrier I hadn't even noticed was there until it lifted – that made me wonder what function that barrier was serving.

I step outside and take a breath as I try to ground myself. There's a lot of bollocks that gets said about grounding. We're told that we can buy things to ground ourselves – face scrubs, candles and bracelets – but grounding means observing the sheer fact of our connectedness with the world and the properties we share with everything around us. Certain contemplative practices can help us with that observation.

As I breathe, and prepare myself to head back into the meditation hall, I notice the sun on my skin and imagine the density of the bones in my feet, not separate from the soles of my shoes, not separate from the paving stones as solid as the distant mountains and the soil underneath me. The soil packed full of worms that are squidgy just like me, and roots that hold up the columns of the trees, that hold up the canopy that dapples the sun onto my skin.

I raise my face towards the light and look into the pink static of my eyelids. I notice a new sensation stirring in my chest that seems to have come out of nowhere and seems to have something to say.

Escapist

In 1940, my grandfather André Bretécher was conscripted from his job as a legal clerk in Nantes into the French army, leaving behind his pregnant wife, Yvonne. He was captured and imprisoned for five years in a Nazi labour camp, escaping in 1945, just months before the end of the war. Arriving home, André met his daughter, Claire, now 5 years old, who would grow up to become one of France's most beloved artists. In the aftermath of the war, André and Yvonne had a second daughter, my mother, who would one day find her way to England's Midlands, where she would meet my dad. Having drunk only water throughout his imprisonment (hell for a Frenchman), my Papy André vowed, save for his morning coffee, to only ever drink wine again. He kept the vow. Mom said he never spoke about the war.

Threshold

'We have a biography, which precedes our mentality and the inner psychological biography of our minds . . . There is a longing within you, which is not just your own.'[1]

John O'Donoghue, poet

I looked out of the car window at the grey water of the Liffey and scanned the banks for kingfishers and herons. Optimistic, I know, on a busy, grey Dublin day, but when you've got twitching in your blood, you always have half an eye on the birds. I used to be a member of the Young Ornithologists' Club, the youth wing of the Royal Society for the Protection of Birds, which makes it sound more fascist than it was, since we mostly counted garden birds. Though there's plenty of politics at the bird feeder.

Every year our family would go to Slimbridge to watch the wildfowl flocks arrive from Africa. Once we travelled to Skomer Island to see the puffins in nesting season. Mom had big '90s hair then. Dad wore a leather bomber. I hold a snapshot in my mind of Dad in that jacket, binoculars around his neck, cheerfully slipping on a steep grass bank and Mom grinning next to him, her hair all over the place in the Welsh sea wind.

I was in the back of a taxi with a podcast producer, the two of us travelling from Dublin Airport to Trinity College Dublin. We were on our way to the Institute of Neuroscience to interview a scientist about mental health diagnoses.

'How was your meditation retreat?' she asked.

'It was amazing. Yeah, it was . . . I learned so much.'

I trailed off through a series of platitudes. I didn't even mention the altered state, the insights from which had already faded in the two months since. Insights tend to do that when you have no way to concretise and ritualise them, no framework to hang them off, no container to hold them. My OCD was fucking terrible. I didn't tell her that either, since she'd already told me that my story of recovery had meant so much to her. I didn't want to let her down.

Now that my book had been out a couple of years, I found myself part of an active community of mental health advocates. Every day I would chat with sufferers and therapists from all over the world and regularly participate in talks and panels and media appearances. In the crowded hallways of conferences, I often found myself embracing strangers and learning intimate details about their lives. It never felt weird or too much, because in some ways, thanks to our shared battle with OCD, we already knew each other. The affection and solidarity reinforced the legitimacy of the story that brought us there, the campfire that we gathered around: mental illness.

When you internalise a story and you live it alongside others in community, that story becomes an identity. The more I felt I belonged, the more the story baked in, and continuing to share in that belonging subconsciously meant sticking to the central tenets of our story, the messages we received from charities, advocates and psychs and repeated back to each other, in a constantly reaffirming loop:

mental illnesses are illnesses like any other;
mental illnesses are caused by biological problems in the brain;
mental illnesses indiscriminately affect 1 in 4 people in the world.

I was accustomed to having this world view reflected back at me in softball media engagements about mental health stigma, and I expected more of the same at Trinity. We arrived on campus and were greeted at the doors of the Institute of Neuroscience by Dr Claire Gillan, an affable Irish professor no older than me. Concentration was difficult. While Dr Gillan welcomed us, my mind produced a kaleidoscope of things that I could have done right then that'd get me arrested. I could lose control of my limbs and assault someone. I could spontaneously take all of my clothes off. The thoughts were sticky. They followed me like gum on my shoe through the corridors of the institute – the concrete walls of which I imagined caving in on top of me – and into an office lined with papers and files.

Dr Gillan was using computational modelling and large-scale online data collection to identify 'trans-diagnostic markers of psychiatric disturbances'.[2] In other words, studying a wide range of feelings and behaviours in large numbers of people, regardless of the mental health diagnosis they'd been given. To start the interview, I asked her what she'd discovered.

'OCD is not a biological reality,' Dr Gillan said, very matter of fact.

I felt instant resistance. Something in my chest twisted.

She continued: 'That's what the data are increasingly showing. There are many commonalities when we average across people with OCD. But they are, one, never applicable on an individual basis; and two, not unique to OCD versus other disorders. Inside a single diagnostic category, you see massive variability not only in presentation, but in aspects of brain structure and function.'[3]

I struggled with this information. The friction in my chest was intensifying. I fumbled for a response. What about all the research that'd already been done? Hadn't people already proved that OCD brains are different biologically? (Some neuroimaging studies on people with OCD show increased activity in the basal ganglia, prefrontal cortex and anterior cingulate cortex[4] – my advocate peers were always posting images of brain scans showing a 'normal brain' vs an 'OCD brain'.)

'Abnormalities in these regions are by no means exclusive to OCD,' Dr Gillan explained. 'A great many disorders show the same kinds of brain changes.'

I didn't know this. I'd thought that my brain had the same abnormalities as everyone else with a diagnosis of OCD and that these abnormalities were the root cause of our obsessions;

that we had brains that were reliably and measurably different from the brains of people with, say, depression or anorexia. I had thought that this was the definition of mental health diagnosis. Dr Gillan explained that, on the contrary, when a clinician makes a mental health diagnosis, they're not leaning on any biological data, it's a much more subjective decision.

To be clear, when I question, in this book, the idea that my suffering was a result of a brain disorder, I don't doubt that when we are chronically depressed or anxious or obsessive, activity is happening in our brains that might correlate with our distress. But we don't understand these correlations. It's not like looking at, for example, kidney stones on a scan, where you're literally seeing the source of the pain. As you'll hear Dr Gabor Maté explain to me later, everything we do, from walking, to talking, to falling in love, involves changes in brain activity. When my mental health was at its worst, there would undoubtedly have been changes in brain activity that could be called disordered. But would that brain activity have been causal of my suffering or reflective of it? Arguably both, since our brains change in a use-dependent way, meaning the way we use our brains shapes the way we use them in the future. But that still begs the questions: how, and why, does the brain come to tread these paths in the first place? What accounts for the disorderedness? The overwhelming focus of mental health research in the last half century has been on changing the way the brain is, rather than on the environmental adversities that might lead the brain to become how it is. In any case, what I was reluctantly learning in Dublin is that just because I had a diagnosis of OCD, doesn't mean my brain would necessarily have looked the same as anyone who shared my diagnosis; and that even as descriptions of symptoms, diagnoses are woolly, overlapping and heterogenous.

'Take schizophrenia,' Dr Gillan said, 'where two people can have the same diagnosis but none of the same symptoms. Or depression, where you need five out of nine symptoms on a list of criteria to be diagnosed, meaning there are a couple of hundred combinations of symptoms that a person can present with. It's one of the quirks and flaws in the system we're using to diagnose people.'

Dr Gillan had included in her studies people who have no diagnosed mental health conditions. What she found in an online study of two thousand 'mentally healthy' people, was that many display a variety of traits typically associated with clinical diagnoses, such as compulsivity, anxiety, and social withdrawal, pointing to a spectrum of emotional difficulties in all of us, not just those of us with a clinical diagnosis.

As Dr Gillan kept talking, I felt a skin-crawling aversion. Something in my chest was pulsing, like a far off part of me shouting. But when I focussed on it, my attention was snatched away almost immediately by a flurry of intrusive thoughts.

~

As we crossed the grey waters of the Liffey once more, back over the bridge towards Dublin airport, I didn't notice how the light played on the river. Or if the gulls were managing to fly in the strong winds. I didn't register the shape of the car seat in front of me, though I was staring straight at it. I was off somewhere else, ruminating.

So much of my sense of self and my career was structured around the idea of mental illness. How could I square that with what I'd just heard, about diagnoses not representing biological differences; or discrete categories not pointing to any biological root causes; about there being no biological distinction between the 'ill' and the 'well'?

These findings felt like an attack on the legitimacy of my suffering. Like I'd been told it wasn't real. Like people were doubting the seriousness or validity of my problems. Without realising, I was falling for what psychologist Mary Boyle has identified as the false 'brain or blame dilemma'[5]: the fear that unless we are seen as having an illness with a label, others will blame us for our distress, or otherwise assume that our distress is not 'real'. I pressed my fingernails into my palms in feeble frustration. I wasn't making it up! I'd been told I had a literal illness by people in suits with letters after their names.

There was one reader letter I'd received way back in 2013, from a woman in her fifties who'd secretly been experiencing the same intrusive thoughts as me her whole adult life. She'd put my article in the lap of her elderly mother and said, 'Mum, this is me. I've got OCD'. They'd hugged each other and wept. That's what diagnosis meant to me.

We arrived at the airport and walked into the endless day of the flood-lit departures hall. In the customs queue I took my phone out.

Google
Vuklogical roop
Crap

Backspace
Biological root causes for mental health diagnoses
Search

It's embarrassing to think that, as a mental health advocate and a supposedly curious and educated person, I'd never thought to ask this question before. Mental illnesses as biological illnesses was just *how things were.* I'd never questioned whether gravity was real either.

I read a little, then shuffled in the queue. Read, shuffle, read, shuffle. It was quickly apparent that Dr Gillan's findings were not anomalous, they were in keeping with innumerable critiques of the scientific dubiousness of mental health diagnosis dating back years, from leading academics at universities I'd heard of. It seemed there was a decades-old debate about not only the validity of diagnosis but the entire philosophy of treating distress as illness. Apparently, a guy called Thomas Insel, the director of the National Institute of Mental Health (NIMH) in America, had said that the search for biomarkers that upheld discrete psychiatric diagnosis had been fruitless.[6] This seemed like a big deal, which confused me further. Why had I never heard about this? I felt aversion and curiosity at the same time. The urge to investigate and the urge to stick my fingers in my ears.

I got through customs to the between-land of the departure lounge. I looked in the shops for something to stave off the discomfort of being neither here nor there. I bought an eye mask and earplugs, to not see and not hear. I watched a one Euro coin spiral into a wishing well. I drank a so-so coffee. I walked down the jet bridge that stretched between

41

the plane and the terminal, lost between stories. As I fastened my seatbelt, I could feel the side of my arse touching that of my neighbour. The tannoy said we could expect turbulence.

As the plane took off, people reached for magazines and headphones and miniature cans of G&T to kill time before the piss light came on in about twenty minutes. No wifi up here. No choice but to sit in your cognitive dissonance.

That fucking knot in my chest again. *What do you want?* Pulsing like an alarm.

I focussed on the sensation and was almost immediately distracted by the warm dough of my neighbour's arse.

Back to the sensation.

Then distracted by a narrow jet of aircon that smelled like kitchens.

Back to the sensation.

Then distracted by a thought of eating my neighbour out . . .

Back to the sensation.

You can time travel when you do this: go back to your body again and again until it lets you in, follow your sensations like a thread, a *tantra*, into the past, dropping back to the last time you felt them. With my feet safely grounded on the floor of the plane, I closed in on the pulsing density of the knot and my thoughts emerged a couple of hours earlier in Dr Gillan's office, the last time the alarm had been triggered:

'OCD is not a biological reality,' Dr Gillan said, very matter of fact. I felt instant resistance. Something in my chest twisted.

Why was my aversion to this fact so strong? What was that twisting? The answer wasn't here in this memory. It was somewhere else, a little further back in time. As Gillan keeps talking, notice the solidity of that chest knot, how it seems to get denser at the core, and follow its thread 2000 miles across the Atlantic and eight weeks further into the past, up through the sandy Californian soil, through a grey carpeted floor and into a meditation retreat, where I had just emerged from a non-ordinary state of consciousness.

I raised my face towards the light and looked into the pink static of my eyelids. I noticed a new sensation stirring in my chest that seemed to have come out of nowhere and seemed to have something to say.

As I had waited to go back into the meditation hall, I'd tried to pay attention to this new sensation. It was intensely unpleasant and nauseating, pressing on my chest and up into my throat; a dense snarl of energy the size of a fist. It was mysterious – somewhere between an emotional feeling and a physical feeling. If it'd had a colour, it would've been dark. If it'd had a temperature, it would've been hot. Like a lump of coal burning my flesh from the inside. It felt new, but also somehow old. Bizarrely and eerily I knew immediately that this sensation had been here my whole life, I just hadn't ever noticed it. Like it was a frequency that had always been broadcasting but I'd only now tuned in. Like it had always been down there in the murkiness of what the Buddha called 'the fathom-long body'[7] and had only just surfaced.

More bizarrely, I noticed that I could only feel this emotional knot on the left side of my throat. The right side of my throat, in fact the right side of my whole body, was relatively numb and devoid of sensation, like the dark side of the moon. How can something be happening in your body, or in half your body, your entire life without you knowing? And why had it only emerged now in the wake of a mystical experience?

Back then, I had not encountered the theory that a person can carry fragments of emotions from a very long time ago and that these can resurface as inexplicable physical sensations. I hadn't heard about the idea of body memories or emotional flashbacks, or about the theory that trauma affects the left and right hemispheres of your brain differently. I didn't know that this was the first foothold of a long and difficult climb back into bodily sensations I'd once been too vulnerable to feel. All I knew, as I stood bewildered and sceptical on that persistently strange day, was that a Gordian knot of emotion had just announced its lifelong residency in my chest.

Above a treeline of Californian sugar pines, the birds of prey were still flying, resting and rising through invisible thermals in the cloudless air. Follow those currents up and up to 30,000 feet above the Irish Sea, two months later, where my new–old sensation that had resounded like a klaxon in Dr Gillan's office just hours before, now seemed to be telling me something: listen. There was something salient about your aversion to what she'd said: listen. *My internal life had been marked by doubt, but this intuition was clear: listen.*

~

THUD. I dropped my medical records onto the kitchen table.
CRACK. I pulled my knuckles and readied myself for a deep dive.

I traced my fingers down the pages to find the diagnoses I'd been given over the years: obsessive compulsive disorder, depression, generalised anxiety disorder, premenstrual dysphoric disorder, bulimia. Each one of these labels represented a painstaking assessment process that had involved me delivering my opening gambit about my intrusive thoughts, filling in forms, getting referred, repeat, check-up, repeat.

I flipped the pages and saw references to the methods of investigation (stethoscopes, phlebotomy, blood pressure pumps, X-rays, otoscopes) that'd yielded very reliable data about my other health problems. On the day that I was born, for example, doctors had quickly and accurately determined the cause of the red rash on my arse and applied a targeted treatment. It sounds obvious to say this, but I realised that by contrast, my psychiatric diagnoses had never involved any objective tests. I'd taken on these diagnoses as if they were biological explanations of my problem, but I realised with a facepalm that they'd been based solely on what I'd said about my feelings and experiences. And what I said wasn't a fixed thing – it would change depending on how I was understanding myself at any given time.

I was confused by something I'd read at the airport: that no one had ever found a biological root cause for any mental health diagnosis. There was no gene or collection of genes. No pathogens. No changes in tissue growth or structure. I assumed this couldn't be true: otherwise, what was our entire mental health system based on? How could my illness be like any other, but not testable like any other, definable like any other or treatable like any other? I realised I hadn't thought through, let alone interrogated, the messages that I was spreading in my advocacy. I'd often cited statistics from the World Health Organization in my public speaking and now found myself questioning what those stats meant. When the WHO categorised mental health conditions according to the International Classification of Diseases (ICD) and calculated the contribution of these conditions to 'the global burden of disease',[8] what did they mean by 'disease'? Were they saying I had one? Or, as my health records implied, had I had many separate ones? Or, as psychiatry's critics claimed, was mental disease more a fictional paradigm than a factual one? I'd left California wondering how the symptoms of mental illness can suddenly and absolutely subside. I hadn't so much answered it as evolved the question: was mental illness even the right framing?

'Where had one [diagnosis] ended and the others begun? I couldn't make narrative sense of it,' I wrote at the time. 'I still need to make sense of what I've been through. I need a concept. I need a story. So how else can I conceptualise mental health? Perhaps not as a suite of self-contained conditions, stacked in the past like shoeboxes, but something that's still moving. A shoal of fish: a million traits, experiences, impressions and impulses – washing past each other, interacting at innumerable points . . . Sometimes they wind tightly into giant arrows or daggers. Sometimes they dissipate and let the sunlight through. The lack of containment in this conception of mental health unsettles me. To resist a neatly-drawn distinction between personality and pathology is frightening – as a human being I want boundaries, some way to hem in and package up the nightmare. But in its fluidity, it is also comforting. It lets me off the hook: no more need to put the bad bits in a box called "disorders" and the good bits in a box called "me".'

~

Integration is the bringing together of separate elements into a whole. To integrate a psychological or ideological shift, new material needs to be assimilated into the context of your life. When babies experience big emotions, their caregivers will instinctively reflect those emotions back at them. Securely attached mothers will screw up their faces when their babies do, and pout when their babies do. This shows the baby that what's going on inside has a place in the context of the wider world. *Look! Your feelings are okay because they are embodied out here.* As grown-ups we continue to need our minds reflected back at us. Our loved ones will subconsciously mirror our faces when we talk, giving us canvasses on which we can see our inner lives projected, making us feel less alone. I didn't see my tentative scepticism of the medical model mirrored back at me in any public conversation I was part of.

I remember the moment that I ironically started to feel stigmatised by the diagnostic framework that I'd promoted as destigmatising. I'd been commissioned by one of the broadsheets to write an article about my life with OCD. I'd incorporated in the piece some of the questions that meditation had raised about the blurred boundaries between what we call illness and what we call self. The editor cut all of this context and came back with a paragraph-by-paragraph brief: define OCD, list its symptoms, explain how you overcame these symptoms. It was hard to find a way to talk about mental health at all without using medical language. Diagnosis seemed to be the load-bearing wall that made conversation possible.

I certainly didn't see my scepticism mirrored back at me by mental health care, where no doctor ever explained what diagnosis did and didn't mean. Neither did I see it in advocacy, where my peers continued to follow our familiar formula:

more awareness raising =
more funding for research into biological root causes =
more people receiving correct diagnoses =
more people accessing the targeted help they need.

I tried to wear two hats at first, continuing to follow the formula in public while questioning its soundness in private. I found the critical psychiatry literature fascinating, and that fascination allowed me to keep the material at a distance. Questioning the medical paradigm was an intellectual pursuit that did not necessarily mean joining my emotional dots. But cognitive dissonance always gets you in the end.

~

In early 2018, the Channel 4 adaptation of *Pure* began filming on the streets of London. The first time I went down to set it was a stormy, snowy night. The medic had had to pay special attention to a bus full of naked extras to prevent hypothermia.

I walked down Old Street to the shoot location in Shoreditch. This neck of the woods was where I'd come of age. It held memories of chaotic nights out, people I'd known, mistakes I made, bars I'd worked behind. I turned the corner at Shoreditch Church and looked down the high street to see sixty-odd people in high-vis vests and kit vans and an entire film crew. All assembled to bring *Pure* to life.

Later in the shoot, in an old academic library, we filmed a romanticised version of the moment I first discovered that intrusive thoughts were a symptom of a condition called OCD, a moment of feeling seen, of the world finally making sense. In one of the more meta moments of my life, actor Charly Clive wept in front of the camera as I wept behind it – watching, as well as living, the story that had started in my heart a long time ago, which was supposed to be over but was still tearing me apart.

As the action played out in take after take, I took a seat halfway up a spiral staircase. The cold steel spiralled down to where I'd just come from and up to another part of the library I hadn't explored. The dramatic irony of watching this supposed turning-point moment with a head full of intrusive thoughts that were as bad as ever? I couldn't process it.

By early 2019, with the buzz of the show, the sense of professional achievement, and the financial boost it'd given me, I was feeling less anxious. I watched the live broadcast with my family and friends on a big screen. We shouted and screamed. It was a-rolling-around-laughing-on-the-floor kind of evening, which turned into an early morning, which turned into a late morning, which turned into an empty seat in a BBC studio where I was supposed to be being interviewed live on Radio 4 but completely missed my slot. With a cracking hangover and a heartful of last night's well wishes, I called up my mate to ask if he'd tuned in for my no-show and we laughed. There were times like this, even when I was very sick, when I knew that I was lucky to be alive and that somehow everything was going to be okay, because I wouldn't stop until it was.

Repeat beats

'To exist is to change, to change is to mature, to mature is to go on creating oneself endlessly.'[1]

Henri Bergson, philosopher

When poet John Donne, the dean of St Paul's Cathedral, ambled up the pulpit steps in 1631, he knew this would be his last sermon, so he made sure God could hear him. Clouded in incense and lit by candlelight, the dying man trembled as he thundered out a ferocious hour-long contemplation on death to his riveted congregation. 'There in the womb we are fitted for works of darkness, all the while deprived of light,' he boomed, 'and there in the womb we are taught cruelty, by being fed with blood, and may be damned, though we be never born.'[2]

With wide eyes I read these fantastically grisly words centuries later. Donne's writing, which as a teenager I'd newly discovered, was feverish, passionate, tender, morbid, devotional. He wrote about love, death, separation, lust, and seduction. I hung a poster of him on my wall. To be fair, he was very much my type: a tortured artist with a gift for the gab. I had a history of falling in love with unavailable men and it didn't get more unavailable than a centuries-dead clergyman.

When he died, Donne didn't know that a piece he'd written years before would become one of the most famous in all of literature: 'No man is an island, entire of itself, every man is a piece of the continent, a part of the main . . . and therefore never send to know for whom the bell tolls, it tolls for thee.'[3]

I didn't know as a teenager that the same piece would crop up again and again in the trauma literature I'd later immerse myself in, cited by authors exploring human inter-connectedness and the inextricable ties between our stories. We are all united in this shared life, Donne was saying. The same bell (the funeral bell), tolls for all of us.

But Donne's last sermon was not so much about death, as about change. Donne characterises change as the constant passing away of moments. 'In all our periods and transitions in this life, are so many passages from death to death,' he said to the congregation of St Paul's. 'Our birth dies in infancy, and our infancy dies in youth, and youth and the rest die in age, and age also dies and determines all.' In a blood-curdling image, he warns us of what happens if we try to resist the inevitability of change: 'Neither is there any grave so close or so putrid a prison, as the womb would be to us if we stayed in it beyond our time.'[4] If we refuse to be born into the next moment, the comfort we cling to will destroy us.

Donne had never encountered Buddhism, but ideas like this had been percolating in Asia for two millennia. In Buddhist traditions, paradoxically, flux is our only certainty and the constant death of moments is our definition of life. 'Everything changes' is how Japanese Zen monk Suzuki Roshi describes the Buddha's most basic teaching.[5] It is also the most basic teaching of storytelling.

~

Screenwriters pace their work with beats, the smallest unit of change in a story. Each beat of the story pushes the protagonist's emotional arc forward in a new way. A new motivation. A twist of fate. A lesson learned. A story with beautifully orchestrated beats feels so alive we temporarily inhabit its life, quite forgetting our own. When there are too many 'repeat beats' – i.e. the events surrounding a character are changing, but their emotional arc is not – stories start to drag. We don't have to study anything about stories to recognise this, we're born with the knowledge. We sense repeat beats instinctively and with no effort. Our bodies might start fidgeting or sighing, as if by filling our lungs we might also oxygenise what's happening on screen. We feel good stories in our bodies because stories speak *change*, the language of our bodies. If a story stops embodying change, we sense it. If we stop feeling the essential ebb and flow of thresholds resisted and then crossed, the story is lifeless.

In the wake of the *Pure* broadcast in early 2019, the village that had sprung up around me, in which there was always something to do, someone calling on me, some mutual accountability or engagement to make, disappeared. I don't know why I did what I did, but I watched myself go to the pharmacy, buy razors, take them home and cut the skin of my thighs. I looked down at my body, that had sat like this, feeling numb like this, with my arms holding my knees in close like this, on a different bathroom floor in a different decade, and realised nothing had changed, nothing had progressed. This body was reenacting the same beat of the story again and again, treading the same old ground with the same old maps. Again, this. I went to sleep and had the same recurring nightmares I'd had since I was a child. I woke up to an inbox full of people seeking advice about how to live.

Pure went around the world, bringing new waves of interest with each new territory. And as I literally watched my old story diffusing around me, the pressure of a new, untold and much scarier story was starting to build. Accompanied by just the faintest outline of a question that I had been trying to keep down. That I wouldn't be ready to face until psyche-delic drugs broke me down into bits and then put me back together again. If illness wasn't the root cause of my suffering, what was?

PART TWO

Confrontation

'The pain recurs again and again, until the desire to take out that thorn is constantly with you. In the end, it reaches a point where you make up your mind once and for all to get that splinter out because it hurts . . . Wherever it hurts, wherever there's friction, we must investigate. Confront the problem head on. Take that thorn out of your foot . . . Wherever suffering arises, look into it. Look right into the present moment. Look at your own mind and body. When suffering arises, ask: why is there suffering? Look right now.' [1]

Ajahn Chah,
Thai Buddhist monk

Philosopher's stones

'The madness is calling us to the Gods . . . either as a frenzy
or as a love or as a ritual initiation into a new kind of life.'[2]

James Hillman, psychologist

2017

A diagram of a circle. Inside the circle, lots of coloured lines
overlap each other. The image represents what happens to
the brain on psilocybin, the psychoactive compound in magic
mushrooms. The lines are illustrative of the increased connectivity and novel pathways between brain networks that the
drug seems to carve. A second circle to the left, representing
the brain on placebo, is sparse, less colourful and comparatively drab.

These twin circles, and the 'before and after' story they
imply, have become a symbol of the psychedelic renaissance
– a resurgence of mainstream interest in psychedelic
compounds beginning in the 2010s, which had originally

waned when LSD was made illegal in the UK in 1966 and psilocybin in 1971. These twin circles would be used on the inside sleeve of journalist Michael Pollan's *How to Change Your Mind*, the bestselling book of the renaissance.[3] They were being presented on a big projector screen by neuropsychopharmacologist Professor David Nutt of Imperial College London, who I'd come to see give a talk about psychedelics research.

There were some quite hot men there: utilitarian clothes, tortoiseshell-glasses types, lots of smart watches. My seat was quite far back, so I could mainly just see the sides of jawlines, the backs of well-barbered necks and people's social feeds on their phones. We got a free drink on entry but I finished mine before I sat down.

Since my altered state of consciousness in California, I'd been curious to learn of some researchers' speculation that psychedelics and long-term meditation practice might do something similar to the brain.[4] Maybe learning about psychedelics could help me understand what my sober trip was, and what could account neurobiologically for the sudden, brief cessation of my mental illness?

The term 'psychedelic' was coined in 1957 by British psychiatrist and LSD researcher Humphry Osmond. It means 'mind manifesting'[5], from the Greek *psykhē* (mind/soul) and *dēloun* (to make visible, reveal), and the Proto-Indo-European root *dyeu* (to shine). Osmond was the doctor who first gave mescaline, a cactus-derived psychedelic, to writer Aldous Huxley, a trip that Huxley wrote about in *The Doors of Perception*. Like many people, when I read the book I felt the tracing of an aesthetic line from his trip to mine, from psychedelics to meditation and back again, through the semantic field of what both can feel like: bright, shining, shimmering.

Huxley called his expanded state of consciousness on mescaline, 'Mind at Large', in which the mind is able to perceive details in the environment that are usually edited out as useless. 'To make biological survival possible,' he wrote, 'Mind at Large has to be funnelled through the reducing valve of the brain and nervous system. What comes out at the other end is a measly trickle of the kind of consciousness which will help us to stay alive on the surface of this particular planet.'[6]

Huxley, Buddhist mystic Ram Dass and English writer Alan Watts were among several twentieth-century scholars leading the translation of the wisdom of ancient and eastern traditions to Western psychonauts. Huxley was saying that, normally, we don't perceive the world as it is, we perceive the mind's reconstruction of the world, a construction that permits us to see only what is necessary, not what is beautiful or surprising. So when we think we're looking at a tree, we're not actually seeing a tree as it is, we're seeing a functional representation of a tree compressed through a reducing valve.

The audience at David Nutt's talk was very middle class, mostly white. And very *media*. The man in front of me spent most of the time taking photos, editing them, and posting them to Instagram. I think it would be fair to say that the main reason he was there, and that everyone else was there, in the plush auditorium of that private members club, writing notes in their Moleskines and sipping mezcal cocktails, was because they are WEIRD: Western, Educated, Industrialised, Rich, and Democratic. As psychedelics researcher Rayaan Zafar would explain to me years later, it's not just the renaissance punters who are WEIRD, it's the people on whom the studies are conducted. The acronym was coined in reference to the sampling bias in Western psychological research, which tends to study college students and those in academia, who are not only unrepresentative of humans as a species, but are also outliers on many psychological measures, tending to be more materially privileged and individualistic and less bound by tradition. WEIRD people represent as much as 80 per cent of study participants, but only 12 per cent of the world's population. This becomes a problem if treatments (i.e. psychedelic therapy), which are tested on these populations, are then assumed to be helpful for humans generally. If, like most of the world, you experience financial deprivation and lack of access to education, or if you live anywhere but in a rich Western democracy, your experiences are not being captured by the kind of research that was being presented tonight.

Professor Nutt had been fired in 2009 from his position as drugs policy advisor to the UK government for declaring that ecstasy is statistically safer than horse riding. He wrote a satirical paper outlining the harms of horse riding called 'Equasy: An overlooked addiction with implications for the current debate on drug harms'.[7]

The neuroscience, Nutt was saying as he pointed at the twin circles, seems to track with the phenomenology, i.e. with what people say about their psychedelic experiences. When psilocybin is taken at high doses (with the right mindset and in a supportive setting) it not only seems to promote novel and diverse connections in the brain, it also seems to enable people to think about their problems in new ways and overcome negative thought loops. Nutt's colleague at the time, Professor Robin Carhart-Harris, compares these effects to shaking a snow globe; to the temporary chaos that enables the brain to settle in a new way like fresh powder after a blizzard. I was struck by this idea of connectivity and how similar it sounds to creativity. It sounded like these drugs have the same integrative action as metaphors themselves: they bring disparate elements together so that novel meaning can emerge. Novelty can be a threat to a hyper-controlled psychic system like mine, and honestly, I was nervous as hell even listening to this stuff. I could feel the tension sitting in my throat.

I've always been nervous about the idea of drugs, even when I was taking them regularly. I was the person who chipped in twenty quid, never the person who got into the dealer's car. The drugs I took in my teens, twenties, and early thirties were illegal. That means that they are considered wrong by the most powerful people in the country. All drug-taking happens within this atmosphere of moral judgement, which has a way of seeping through the living room walls of private citizens and sitting heavily, if subconsciously, on their minds. It puts angels and devils on our shoulders – *this is fun but it is bad, I want it but I shouldn't* – and creates an unhelpful counter dynamic whereby rebels say yes and fuddy-duddies say no. It's hard to escape this context. Even if you believe, as I do, in each person's right to freely alter their consciousness as long as they're not harming others, you're not above it. Our society is permeated with the idea that psychoactive chemicals are inherently immoral, sinful, dirty and dangerous. We breathe it in.

In 1995, an 18-year-old British girl called Leah Betts died after drinking seven litres of water while on ecstasy. Officially she died of water intoxication that made her brain swell. She drank too much water too quickly, much more than her body could process. This may have been exacerbated by ecstasy's inhibition of normal urination. The frenzied trial by media that followed made much of the latter and overlooked the former, deciding almost unanimously: ecstasy killed Leah Betts. When I was in secondary school, Leah's father came to talk to the pupils about drugs. He told the heartbreaking story of his daughter's death. He played us an anti-drugs campaign video. He showed us a picture of his daughter in a coma, shortly before she died, with tubes coming out her nose and her mouth hanging open. Many of us wept as he spoke. He asked us how many of us we thought would be offered drugs by the time we were 18.

A few kids shouted out guesses: 50 per cent? 70 per cent?

He shook his head. 100 per cent, he said. By the time we were 18, all of us would have been offered drugs. The message was unequivocal: drugs kill, say no.

Meanwhile there was no mention of the drug which, at the age of 14, all of us had already sculled from plastic bottles on park benches or sipped merrily from our parents' glasses at Christmas. One study that analysed the extent to which various substances cause harm (dependence, impairment of mental functioning, death, crime, economic cost and impact on family life, etc.) found that alcohol was eight times more harmful than MDMA and twelve times more harmful than psilocybin.[8]

And yet, though it's very rare, people do die from taking ecstasy. To honour the seriousness of this risk we can do things like educate young people about how to minimise harm, provide free drug testing facilities so that people can verify exactly what they're taking, and circulate 'flight instructions' that offer guidance on how to handle challenging drug experiences.

It's also true that mushrooms can break fragile minds. When we were still at school, a best friend of ours took magic mushrooms at a house party, had a devastating trip, and in his own words 'went completely fucking crazy'. In the aftermath, a darkness came over him that lasted for years. He suffered paranoia, anxiety and sleeplessness. He wasn't the same person, to himself or his friends. He'd been taken by the doom drugs we'd heard whispers about in the playground. This is exactly what we'd been educated to do: strip the drug of any context, demonise it and therefore be too frightened to take it. We concluded that magic mushrooms were a guaranteed gateway to psychological hell and vowed we would never do them ourselves.

My ears pricked up when David Nutt said that people who feel stuck in the past, people with *trauma* – that word was coming up a lot – often seem to find themselves getting unstuck after taking psilocybin. I made a note and went back over it several times until the lines were thick with ink.

I was thinking back to what Professor Gillan had said in Dublin just two weeks before, about many traits cutting across diagnostic lines, and how, now that I thought about it, almost everyone I've ever spoken to with a mental health diagnosis describes their problem as some kind of stuckness. 'Getting unstuck' was exactly what seemed to happen in California, when the reducing valve of constricting thoughts had loosened and my mind was briefly at large. When the valve had tightened again, I'd felt the crushing sensation of coming back into my normal reality, and my OCD had been unrelentingly terrible ever since.

My friend, for example, had asked that morning if I wanted to come and work in a cafe rather than work from home. This tiny decision triggered three hours of intense, chest-twisting prevarication, which I tried to counter by making a choice (staying home) and sticking to it. But as I sat down at my desk and tried to work, I repeatedly (once every minute or so) got lost in a mental showreel of what I'd be doing if I'd made the other decision – getting on my bike, cycling to the cafe, speaking to my friend, working in the cafe – trying to verify how that alternate reality compared to this one. My OCD seemed to be tied up with an existential conundrum. Unlike poet Robert Frost as he famously contemplated the two roads which 'diverged in a yellow wood', I could not choose one route or the other. Psychologically, I had to find a way to travel both, even if it tore me apart. For some reason I could not fathom, I always had to be in two places at once.

After the Q&A, there was toe-curling networking chatter – a polite frenzy of *getting*. Getting contacts, getting information, getting pissed. There's lots of reasons why I'm bad at networking, not least because when talking to strangers

I'm always having two conversations: one with them, one with a part of me who is trying to judge me through their eyes. Plus, it's hard to listen to what people are saying when you're concurrently trying to figure out for certain if that thought you just had about fucking them means you want to.

From what I gathered, most people there were 'micro-dosing' on psilocybin, i.e. taking tiny sub-perceptual amounts of it frequently. Anecdotally, some people (mainly tech bros and angel investors, if this crowd was anything to go by) report things like elevated mood and improved focus. I quite like the sound of sub-perceptual effects of low doses, since it's the perceptual effects that I'm so scared of. I was convinced that I had the kind of mind like that of my school friend, one that would get so bent out of shape by a big trip it would never fit back through the door.

(Hypothetically, by the way, if you were a psychedelics rookie who was terrified of psychedelic drugs, but you were inspired by a talk on psychedelics, and you wanted to dip a toe in low doses of psilocybin with a view to one day having a high dose in the hope of curing your chronic mental illness, and you were trying to get your hands on some magic truffles known as philosopher's stones, and you'd decided to order them online, you'd be wise not to get them delivered to your work address.)

INT. POST ROOM - DAY

Rose edges up to the post room hatch. She peeks
through and scans the vast library of letters and
parcels. Hundreds of Amazon faces smile down at her.
The post room attendant, Barry, appears and startles
her.

                    BARRY
          Hi.
                    ROSE
          Hi.

Rose continues scanning the shelves.

                    ROSE
          Did a package arrive for me?

Barry turns to the pigeonholes.

                    BARRY
          Let's see.

Rose smiles nervously. As Barry peruses, she glances
past him into the back room, where a 12-year-old boy
in Bermuda shorts and a tie-dye T-shirt is playing a
Game Boy. They share a smile, a moment interrupted
by:

                    BARRY
          What does the package look like?

                    ROSE
          Er, I don't know.

                    BARRY
          Big? Small?

                    ROSE
          Small, I guess. Discreet.

Barry registers her word choice, which she instantly
regrets. He disappears into a cubby, past the empty
chair where the kid was sat a minute ago but is
now nowhere to be seen. Barry keeps talking
offscreen (O.S.).

                    BARRY O.S.
          It's not in your pigeonhole. It's
          Cartwright, isn't it?

Rose mortifies as she remembers:

                    ROSE
          It's under another name.

                    BARRY O.S.
          What's the name?

Rose looks around sheepishly. A colleague wanders
past and says 'hi'. Rose takes a pen and writes on
a Post-it note. Barry's head emerges impatiently
from the cubby. Rose gestures towards the note.
Barry reads it and shoots Rose a sceptical look.

                    BARRY
          Right. Well that's probably why it
          hasn't been indexed.

Barry goes over to a pile of miscellaneous mail.

                    BARRY
          Is it fragile?

                    ROSE
          No.

                    BARRY
          Perishable?

                    ROSE
              (in silent panic)
          Oh god. Maybe? It's edibles.
          Edible.

                    BARRY
          Right.

Barry turns to have another rummage. Rose nods
apologetically at the couple of colleagues who've
appeared and are forming a queue behind her.

                    BARRY
          Look. All domestic mail comes
          through me so . . .

                    ROSE
          It's from Amsterdam.

A beat as Barry raises an eyebrow. Rose smiles. Barry
slides open a hatch into the next cubicle. He shouts
to someone O.S.

                    BARRY
          Any 'discreet' packages from the
          Netherlands for
              (off Post-it)
          Bootsy Collins.

Out on Rose looking around, laughing nervously.

INT. TOILETS - MINUTES LATER

Rose sits on a toilet, seat down, hastily unwrapping a sorry-looking bundle of bubble wrap. Her frantic hands stop when they uncover a mysterious looking box with a mysterious-looking label:

'Philosopher's stones'

Slowly, she takes out a little lumpy tuber. She holds it up to the light and turns it in her fingers. It looks like it's made of gold.

Magic

'We need a particular form of help at every crucial threshold
. . . And without the robust vulnerability in asking for that
help, we cannot pass through the door that bars us from the
next dispensation of our lives. We cannot birth ourselves.'[1]

David Whyte, poet

2019

The train from London to Oxford raced past woodland and
sunlight flickered on the lids of my closed eyes. The strobing
effect was quite trippy. I had taken a microdose of psilocybin
that morning, but I wasn't high or even micro-high.

I'd been microdosing for a while with no discernible
impact on my mental health. At best, I'd sometimes felt
bright and clear and productive for a couple of hours after
dosing. But caffeine can do that, and it's far more accessible.
I had hoped that microdosing might be my gateway to a
higher dose, but I had learned very little from the experience

so far. Paddling doesn't teach you much about deep sea diving either.

I was on my way to Oxford to do a magazine interview with one of the most influential figures in modern psychedelics research, Amanda Feilding. A drugs policy reformer and an original hippie, an anti-establishment figure and an aristocrat, Amanda is a proponent of art as much as of science. This is the quality that drew me to her, since it strikes me that exploring consciousness is as much an artistic task as a scientific one. Amanda's non-profit, the Beckley Foundation, designs and funds psychedelics research and lobbies the government to reform drug laws. She's led several studies with her colleague, David Nutt.

As the train pulled into Oxford station, I reflected back on the previous eighteen months and the series of events that had challenged my understanding of mental health. My altered state, with its sudden, apparently miraculous cessation of my suffering, had led me to question whether my thoughts were a symptom of disease. My trip to Dublin had made me realise that I had misunderstood the meaning of psychiatric diagnosis. My introduction to psychedelic research had suggested that psychedelics' benefits could cut across diagnostic categories.

Since then, I'd gone into study mode, reading around a series of related topics: psychedelics, meditation, psychology, trauma, critical psychiatry, and consciousness. The story that was unearthed through this reading was huge and difficult to grasp, but very different to the mental illness story I'd grown up with and the one I'd shared in *Pure*, which by now was being watched on TV all over the world. (I knew my star was rising when I was asked to be the ambassador for a brand of thick-gusseted period knickers, which through some unimaginable technology rendered sanitary towels and tampons unnecessary. They offered to pay me in pants.)

The emerging picture from my research looked something like this: common mental health problems were less likely to be a result of organic brain disease and more likely to be a result of environmental stress in the present and the past. Part of me was attracted to this picture, which was less interested in categorising people with mental health problems by their surface differences, and more in the human need for connection that we all share. Part of me had continued to resist it, because it seemed to delegitimise what I'd been fighting for, to be seen as having a 'real' disease, and because on some level I must have known where all of this was heading: to a confrontation with the difficult truths about the stressors of my childhood that I didn't want to face. Turns out, I was very skilled at keeping intellectual knowledge tactically disintegrated from emotional knowledge.

In 2018, I'd gone on my second silent Buddhist meditation retreat. This time it was in the UK, and had a specific focus on working with the body. There I'd started to build a new map of my problem, sinking below the surface layer of compulsive rumination to the actual sensations that my thinking mind was either clinging to or avoiding. It was this piece of the puzzle that I realised I'd been missing, something my psychiatric education had failed to help me understand: that mental health is as much about the body as it is about the brain. There's been a tendency in the West, especially since the seventeenth century when Descartes declared thinking to be the ultimate authority, to try to think our way out of problems and therefore marginalise our embodied nature. 'We have forsaken the body as a source of knowledge,' writes psychologist Stanley Keleman.[2]

Modern life colludes in this abandonment. We have to bury our intuitions to get by. If we want to work, i.e. survive, we have to ignore the stinging in our eyes when the alarm goes off after a fitful sleep; the skin-crawling when we're stuck in traffic; the shudder at the blast of aircon. We are also incentivised to ignore other people's bodies and make ourselves numb to the pleading eyes of the unfortunate strangers we share our cities with.

I had recently read psychiatrist Bessel van der Kolk's book, *The Body Keeps the Score*. No account of mental illness symptoms would resonate for me more than his much broader and more general descriptions of patients who 'feel chronically unsafe inside their bodies', who experience 'gnawing interior discomfort' and are 'constantly bombarded by visceral warning signs.'[3]

In paying attention, on that 2018 retreat, to what was happening in my body while I was worrying, I'd discovered that there were ways of working with physical feelings that are not easily expressed in words, feelings like the mysterious new–old ache in my chest. I'd discovered new senses that I didn't know I had, like interoception (the body's sense of its own internal processes) and proprioception (the body's sense of its location and position in space). I'd discovered sensations of tightness, breathlessness, lightness, warmth, rigidity, trappedness, restlessness, stuckness: a feeling that while everything else was observably changing around me, some-thing inside me was digging in its heels. I would later wonder if the mental illness paradigm was part of the reason I felt stuck, since it fixed an understanding of my problem at a certain point. Interestingly, the etymological roots of 'stuck' and 'stigma' are very similar, meaning to be pierced by a sharp object and unable to move, and to be embedded.

A few months after this latest retreat, there I was, arriving at Beckley Park, Amanda Feilding's moated sixteenth-century mansion in Oxfordshire. I was on a mission to understand my stuckness and wondered if a big dose of psychedelics could set me free.

I was welcomed by staff through the studded Tudor door into a flagstoned sitting room. Every surface was lined with paintings, artefacts, treasures, curios. Amanda entered the room, tall, graceful and charismatic, and we sat in front of the fire.

She leaned in and spoke softly. What brought me here?

I told her how bad things had been and that I was trying to understand what had happened to me.

'It's like there's something locked inside,' I said, placing one hand on my sternum and the other on my throat. 'A physical constriction. Something beyond words. I'm on a personal quest to understand it.'

She nodded. 'Everything I've ever done has started with a personal quest.'

Amanda's fascination with consciousness started young, fed by the romanticism and isolation of Beckley Park – 'it was a kingdom unto itself here' – and by the books on philosophy and psychology her father encouraged her to read. As a teenager, she was the Oxbridge hopeful at her Catholic school and requested books on Buddhism and mysticism from the nuns ('They said "no", I said "bye".'). And at 16 she left England to travel the world: 'I created my own education.'

It wasn't until nine years later, in 1965, that Amanda first took LSD. 'A man who'd become my boyfriend had synthesised it in his kitchen in Ibiza, and after turning the island on, he brought it to the UK.'

What was it like?

'Like a trip to the funfair.'

The experience lit a fire underneath Amanda. She wanted to discover everything she could about consciousness through this new tool.

But by then the moral panic over LSD had begun. The first wave of research in the 1950s and '60s had started to show the therapeutic potential of psychedelics in treating depression, addiction, anxiety and the existential suffering of dying. When the molecules seeped out of the lab and onto the street, they got entangled with the '60s spirit of resistance. 'People went to the park and took LSD with their girlfriends rather than go to a jungle and get shot at. It was considered a threat to the establishment.' The US made LSD illegal in 1968, the UK in 1966.

So Amanda did her own thing, namely four decades of personal experimentation, scientific research and creative collaborations. At 27, while examining the effect of changes in blood flow on consciousness, she famously trepanned herself (drilled a hole in her skull) and filmed it. An audience member fainted during the New York screening of the resulting art documentary, *Heartbeat in the Brain*. As someone who'd just emptied the contents of their mind in a very public way through a TV show, I found myself drawn to

Amanda's method of putting her head at the centre, literally, of her own experiments.

In 1998, Amanda founded the Beckley Foundation, a psychedelics think tank based in the ancient cowhouse next door, which carries out research and lobbies for evidence-based policy reform. 'So I could go into the House of Lords and the UN, like a Trojan horse, armed with science,' she said. Recent studies carried out as part of the Beckley Foundation research programme suggest that psychedelics improve treatment-resistant depression and help people quit smoking. Beckley hopes to see prohibition lifted so that millions can be helped legally in therapeutic settings.

When the coffee and shortbread arrived, I asked Amanda what discoveries her science has uncovered. 'We've shown that psychedelics reduce activity in the Default Mode Network,' she said. The DMN is a collection of hub centres that are thought to work together to control consciousness, policing the amount of sensory information that enters our sphere of awareness. Under trauma, the theory goes, the DMN's hypercontrol works devastatingly well, physically blocking off pathways to pain in an attempt to keep us protected. It suppresses emotion in the moment and in doing so prevents it from being vented in the long term. It regulates, tightens, suppresses.

'That might explain the constricted feeling in your chest,' Amanda suggested. 'Traumas cut paths in the brain, like your trauma has cut a path in yours, that are very deep and difficult to get at.'

I felt a twinge of recognition and swallowed hard.

It's thought that psychedelics may work by disrupting the

DMN's rigidity, reducing its stronghold on the brain and allowing buried information to resurface. This may explain why trippers report accessing and letting go of deep childhood pain. (Psychedelics' reduction of activity in the DMN is the kind of easy-to-understand story that becomes popular through retelling and can ironically become its own kind of default, but there has since been a pivot away from the over-simplicity of this explanatory model.)

Amanda showed me into the Beckley head office, where her team were busy typing at computers. When I enter a new space and meet new people, I'm always subconsciously scanning the room for anything that could upset me. I get a torn feeling of being in two places at once: on the surface, trying to interact with people, and preoccupied somewhere else at the same time. Lightning-quick, my anxiety struck and I had a series of intrusive thoughts of those office-workers naked, so I was relieved when Amanda suggested we take a walk outside.

Amanda uses language creatively and clearly appreciates literature and the spoken word. I wanted to talk to her about the role that language plays in the kind of psychedelic healing she champions. In CBT you're encouraged to use words actively. You rationalise. You change musts to shoulds. You correct false beliefs, as if beliefs were just pieces of language that could be erased if you rubbed hard enough, rather than a complex interplay of emotions and neurobiology. I'm in the business of talk. I idolise words. And yet they've never managed to fully explain or render my most profound and painful experiences. Why?

'Words mean we do all the incredibly brilliant things we do, and also why we're kind of blind, myopic and dangerous,'

Amanda said. 'When a baby is born, their worlds are very fluid. Words haven't got into it yet. It's primal consciousness.' She theorises that, as a baby develops, words like 'no' and 'stop' become enmeshed with the inhibitory conditioning that keeps us from harm ('Stop! Don't touch the stove.') that they're part of a blocking off rather than an opening up.

'So when we started this conversation and I said that something in me felt beyond words, maybe it's physically beyond words?' I asked.

'Yes, that's my theory: prohibitive brain structures become so solid and fixed as they try to protect us. If trauma is very deep, I don't think words can get down to where it's set. Maybe the ways have been blocked off, because it's too dangerous for the psyche to go there.'

For a writer this is a sobering yet liberating thought. The hours of words I've spoken to therapists. Those jotted in scrapbooks. The thousands more I've written as memoirs. Perhaps they could only ever pick at the lock of the door, the wrong tools all this time.

'I think it was Plato who described everyday consciousness as just seeing shadows on the wall of a cave,' Amanda said. In Plato's famous allegory, a group of people have been chained forever inside a cave, looking at shadows on the back wall. With no knowledge of the outside world, they mistake these shadows for reality itself. It's a reminder that the way we model the world in our minds can block us off from seeing things clearly. 'Words form the veils between you and real consciousness,' she added.

When we started talking about the law – if you're caught supplying LSD, MDMA and magic mushrooms, you could get up to life in prison, on a par with rapists and murderers – Amanda grew increasingly animated. 'This devastating barricade of prohibition has caused more suffering to society than almost any other,' she said. 'We have the right of cognitive liberty, so long as it doesn't harm anyone else. The right to do what we like with our own consciousness.'

We talked about the lack of scientific justification for the UK government's drug policy.

'The ruling government is just a projection of the ego in the brain,' Amanda said. 'A person's ego is trying to keep everything under control, and the grip of the government is a projection of that. It doesn't like revolt.'

'The government is our default mode network?' I replied.

'A projection of it, yes.'

Inspired by the neatness of Amanda's metaphor, I shared one I'd been mulling over: 'I was thinking . . . psychedelics destabilise deep-rooted unhelpful systems in the brain. And that's what you've done in your career. It takes a unique and special molecule to disrupt the brain and you're obviously a unique and special person. Your work has been entropic and disruptive, just like psychedelics.'

'Yes, I've been very lucky,' she says. 'I think you're a projection of what's inside. As within, so without, and all that.'

'The tide changed in the 1960s and psychedelic research was shut down,' I said. 'Could it happen again?'

'I don't think so. I think our force has won through.'

We were wrapping up the interview by the time I felt bold enough to ask: 'How do I access therapists who can guide me through psychedelic experiences safely?' The question felt transgressive and the conversation faltered. We were gagged. That's the subtle attack on dignity that authoritarianism achieves – self-censorship. 'I can't get a name, Amanda.'

'I know,' she said.

In the beats of silence that followed, I felt a wash of hopelessness. Maybe the reason that so many psych treatments had failed was because in a part of my psyche, access had been blocked. But I can't find a way into novel psychedelic treatments legally because access is blocked there too. As within, so without.

But Amanda is optimistic that change is coming. Psychedelic-assisted psychotherapy will be part of our near future, Amanda believes. 'When I was a kid, I wanted to water the desert,' she said. 'As I got older I realised the desert was the human brain. That's what we need to water.' She gestured behind us, towards the ancient red-brick building. 'When I tripped here, I saw this house as a red boat in which I could sail the world and hopefully spread happiness. So in a way this has all been the fulfilment of a dream.'

The Beckley Foundation's imaging studies show the birth of new neurons – neurogenesis. Under altered states of consciousness, new dendrons spread out in our brains and new synapses are created, which is thought to open up a critical post-psychedelic period of neuroplasticity during which it's easier for people to find new solutions to old psychological problems. What emerged from my conversation with Amanda was a picture of consciousness that was not fixed and determined, but fluid and buzzing with possibility.

I was raised to think about my suffering as pathology. I was given a semantic field of diseases and cures and pills.

Definitions with hard edges. Maybe I bought into that way of thinking because it gave me discrete linguistic containers – an established framework within which to write and talk. But that framework could not contain my experiences for long.

In the couple of years since the 'sober trip', I'd started to see my mind not as having been faulty but as having tried its best to keep me safe – a shift away from the resentment that the West's illness paradigm had instilled in me. By stopping for the first time in my life to pay attention to consciousness, I'd tripped on an insight: maybe a mind capable of reaching powerfully towards darkness can reach with just as much power in another direction towards something bright. Meditation gave me that intuition. Maybe one day psychedelics can help me know it more fully.

For me, the research at Beckley Park points less to the wonder of psychedelic molecules and more to the wonder of humans. Psychedelics do not work through external alien forces, they seem to harness powerful endogenous mechanisms that have always been inside us, mechanisms which I apparently accidentally sprung in California. As I left Beckley Park, crossing the moat and walking through the old deer grounds towards the road, I was reminded of Stephen King's advice to aspiring writers, which years ago I'd scrawled into my scrapbook: 'Remember, Dumbo didn't need the feather, the magic was in him.'[4]

Night sea journey

'The night sea journey is a kind of *descensus ad inferos* – a descent into Hades and a journey to the land of ghosts somewhere beyond this world, beyond consciousness.'[1]

Carl Jung, psychoanalyst

2019

I push the round, white plate away as I swallow the last nauseous bite of magic truffles. It'll take a little while before things start happening.

I have not been able to find a safe place to do this in the UK. I couldn't get any recommendations from people I know because I don't know the right people. So I have taken a punt on a hippie-looking lady in Amsterdam who advertised her trip-sitting services online. Trip sitters are people who sit with you while you trip. Their main job is to make sure you stay safe and hydrated throughout, and to generally be a supportive presence, especially if the trip goes bad. But there are no standardised guidelines or ethical codes around what that support should and shouldn't look like. You don't need any qualifications to charge people for your trip-sitting services and there is no independent body vetting people for the job. In most countries, the industry is still underground, and therefore risky.

After I'd got the magic truffles, the 'philosopher's stones', delivered to me back in London, I'd recommended the service to a friend. A couple of weeks later he'd got a knock on the door from the border police. Here in Amsterdam, magic truffles are legal, but I can't shake the context of criminality. If you have to leave home to find a safe place to do something legally, you are, in one way or another, on a pariah's journey. I've only told a couple of people back home what I'm doing. Even among my liberal friends and family, psychedelics are misunderstood. I didn't want to add their fear to mine.

The sitter is a wealthy white woman from California called Allison who works in tech. Her partner is here co-facilitating today's session. They have husky, drawn-out voices like YouTube yoga instructors. I wonder if it's tiring to speak like that all the time. They say they do 'energy work', and because they don't offer any specifics about what this involves, I assume it's something that I'm supposed to know, so I don't ask. I look around. There's Buddhist and Hindu iconography everywhere and they play Nepalese choral chant music. It's a nice apartment.

They find that some people like to take a salt bath mid-trip. The essential oils, the warmth of the water and the sensations on the skin, can induce bliss, they've said. I said, 'I don't think I want to do that.' They said I might change my mind once I'm tripping and that they'll run a bath anyway just in case. They say they will 'live DJ' throughout the experience.

Still no effects from the truffles. My anxiety is building.

Allison shows me a deck of oracle cards. On each card is a spirit animal: a bear, a hawk, a turtle and so forth. She asks me to pick a card. These people are kind and I like them and they're trying to help, and today is no day for cynicism. But the cards . . . the sparkly fantasy animals set against mandala motifs and nebulous galaxies, the New Age platitudes in swirly fonts. I can't help but feel disappointed that of all the inspiring art and literature that could be sending me on my way into the unknown, I'm being served the kind of plastic spirituality I've been trying to avoid. I take a card: an owl with fire in its eyes and a crown on its head. 'Ah,' they say. 'This is good.' They say the owl means wisdom and clear-seeing, and that I can use its spirit as a guiding anchor.

There's an exceptionalism around psychedelic drugs that you could call snobbery. An idea that 'classical' psychedelics like psilocybin, LSD and DMT are more spiritual, ceremonial, even 'purer' somehow, than other recreational drugs like meth or crack cocaine. The issue has been brilliantly skewered by Dr Carl Hart, author of *Drug Use for Grown-Ups*[2], who points out that many of those who campaign for psychedelic legalisation continue to demonise less socially sanctioned drugs and their users[3]. This exceptionalism extends, I would say, to the aesthetics that have sprung up around the psychedelic renaissance. I've only just dipped a toe in the 'space' and I'm already growing weary of other people's ideas of what spiritual sounds like: like Max Richter giving Enya a hot stone massage. It's the tonal homogeny that I'm already finding annoying. Ambient electronica. Mystical flute. Gongs. It's all so aggressively *relaxing*. All so *palatable*.

There's one song that I will be destined to hear at every psychedelic gathering, yoga class and pedicure for as long as I live. It's five solid minutes of a woman humming the same soothing phrase. Over and over. Five solid minutes, the same phrase. There's a bit in *The Bell Jar*, when the protagonist can't get the mental image of a dead body out of her mind. 'I felt as though I were carrying that cadaver's head around with me on a string, like some black, noseless balloon, stinking of vinegar.'[4] That's how I feel about this song. Only it stinks of incense instead.

Aesthetics are not trivial. Healing is, in a way, a mission to find external symbols that help us project the complexities inside us. An aesthetic connection with a piece of music, writing, or with art, will allow our feelings to inhabit a bigger arena beyond the structure of our bodies. Psychologist James Hillman, in an entertaining book called *We've Had a Hundred Years of Psychotherapy and the World's Getting Worse*, wrote, 'To get our souls out of the consulting room and out of our private interior space, we need space in the world for the soul's pathology. Then we can relocate the syndromes. The world can then help carry our disorder, for like cures like. Our obsessive ruminations that go on and on, also appear in the repetitive patterns of mosque tiles, friezes and in Celtic manuscripts.'[5]

If we want to project our complexities, sometimes relaxation might not be the goal. We might want to be excited, challenged, energised, frightened, nauseated, even. I would come to know the psychedelic space better, and understand that you don't always have to be safely wrapped up in Brian Eno synths to have a transcendent experience. One of my most formative later trips was not a ceremony at all. It was at a festival on pills listening to eyelash-quivering jungle, where I found myself flooded with wonderful, unholy emotions like drive, appetite and insatiability. It wasn't any less spiritual because the drugs came out of a plastic baggie rather than a ceremonial cup.

As I sit here in this lovely room in Amsterdam, I am buying into a po-faced, jingly-jangly world which is not only financially inaccessible to the community in which I was raised, but also aesthetically and tonally set apart from it. I haven't yet grasped that cultural authenticity is central to healing, and that healing cannot be authentic if it alienates everyone you love.

Everything is slowly starting to sink as the truffles kick in. It's been two years since the awakening of the sensation in my chest with its quiet but insistent 'listen'. Well, I'm listening now.

The first wave of fractals make the room start to sway in my vision. I have a flurry of obsessive thoughts. The veil is trying to zip itself shut.

I take a deep breath in and out.

I won't run from you today.

The thoughts intensify.

Whatever you're holding over the horizon for me you don't need to hold any more. I'm here to see it.

The carpet starts to swim like a rough sea, so I lie down on the couch under a weighted blanket. The trip sitters wish me a fruitful trip and I put on the eye mask.

My hands turn into old people's hands. They are made of meat. They are not part of me.

The universe is pressing on the right side of my skull. I think my skull might break.

My vision is torn in two along the centre by a scorching rip.

I am at the bottom of the universe in a dark oceanic cave. The walls churn and belch. There is no way out. I may be dying.

I am crying more deeply than I've ever cried.

I am in a radiant space of oranges and pinks. My family is here but I don't see them. Each one of their essences is distinct within the same blissful whole.

I'm a little girl in blue pyjamas, waking up from a lovely nap. Someone is tickling the palm of my hand. I am giggling. I stretch out my hands into five-pointed stars.

Classical music moves in droplets. Shapes I've never seen before. I cannot comprehend this beauty. I feel unworthy but the music tells me that I'm worthy. This involves you. You are a part of this.

I hear my mother's cooing French voice. American accents crowd out hers. I wish they would stop talking.

I stir and see that the trip sitters are dancing around the room. I am irritated and disorientated and wretchedly nauseous. Allison helps me to the bathroom door.

In the bathroom I look at myself in the mirror. I see myself both as an old lady and a child at the same time. My face swirls under my touch. Then a voice comes in: 'I love you.' I'm not sure who the 'I' or 'you' refer to, as neither feels like me. The voice continues, beating like a heart: 'I love you now. I loved you then. I loved the idea of you. I love every version of you that could ever have existed. I love everything you could possibly become'. 'I' seemed to start before I was born and extend forever beyond my reality into other would-be realities, into every other potential iteration of me. At the edges of the mirror my face blurs and burns and stretches off to somewhere else.

I might throw up. Allison suggests that I take a salt bath. I want to kick out like a child. I huff and puff as she helps me get my T-shirt off. I say 'no' and put it back on. I get back on the sofa and put my eye mask on.

Another deep wave and I am with Mom. There are no visuals now. Just an atmosphere of her. Diffuse and pristine. She has never not been here and she will never not exist. I can rest safely here.

Then the sense of her starts to fade. I try to catch it with my hands but the more I scramble the more it slips through my fingers. Clouds start to gather in my chest. The pressure is immense. The essence that was her starts to spin into a huge whirlpool in the sky. My chest feels like it's going to break open. I fight and claw but I can't stop the whirlpool getting bigger and darker, taking more of the atmosphere with it, getting quicker and quicker and hurting my chest more and more. I'm screaming, 'Mommy. You can't leave me with this pain in my chest, Mommy', over and over, a hundred times, a thousand times. The essence that was her thins out to a colossal ominous spindle, disappears into a giant black hole in the sky and takes my screaming with it. Then everything snaps to dark and silence.

In that same snap I am suddenly back in the room, bashing my fists against my ears as cacophonous music plays loudly. While tripping I must have manoeuvred my body so that my head was against the speakers. The trip sitters have not realised because they are not in the room. At the sounds of my screams they come rushing back in.

They turn down the music.

They try to talk to me but I stare wordlessly into the middle distance with tears in my eyes. I was with her and now I'm not.

I am desolate and they look worried. They check the clock, I have surfaced hours sooner than expected. So I must still be high.

They don't seem to know what to do.

They ask if they can play me a song that means a lot to them.

I shrug. I have no will. No volition left. I'm not sure if I'm alive.

The song starts. Some violin number that means nothing to me. They are lying on the floor beside the sofa. I see that they are stroking each other's hands as they look at each other and that they have tears in their eyes. It occurs to me that they're high, but I can't trust my perceptions right now.

I write a sentence in my journal, curl up and face away from them.

They ask if I saw the owl.

I shrug.

I ask them to put my music on. A techno track that I love begins, a big banger. It is the sound of rain on concrete and spliffs in the garden with my brother. It is the sound of home. After a long build, the beat drops and kick-starts my heart and I realise my ears can hear this, my body can feel it. My senses mean that I am a part of everything that I sense. As the synths rise, I take my rightful place in this beauty that involves me, and slowly come back to life.

Subplot

'When I think of somebody telling a story, I see a group of people huddled together and around them a vast space, quite frightening . . . In the very idea of the story, there is something to do with shelter . . . this almost physical sense of shelter where the story represents a kind of habitation, a kind of home.'[1]

John Berger, novelist

That evening I lay in my grubby Amsterdam hotel room, looking at the big hairline crack in the ceiling plaster. I don't like cracks because of my structural-integrity-of-buildings obsession.

I shook my head and exhaled as the next wave of bitter disappointment rolled in. My OCD hadn't gone away, nor the pain in my chest. There had been no miracle cures here. It was a small comfort that my intrusive thoughts were now somehow happening in a bigger space, as if my depth of field had altered and brought more of my surroundings into focus.

For a couple of years, I had been consuming information that had challenged the brain–disease paradigm I'd held dear. This information seemed to have been stored in my psyche as blurred, inaccessible bits. Now these bits, and their relationship to my emotional life, appeared clear. All could be viewed within the same integrated frame.

Epiphanies are less a sudden bolt of novelty, more an arrival at a place where a part of you has been waiting for a long time. I'd always known that I'd experienced immense stress in my childhood, but I had, until today, been very successfully burying it.

I'm not going to write in detail about that stress, and most of what happened I won't mention at all. Briefly, my mother's severe bipolar disorder started when I was a baby and returned cyclically for twenty-five years. I watched her get taken away to psychiatric hospital against her will many times throughout my childhood. When she was home, she would spend months in bed with the curtains drawn. I regularly saw and heard things that would have deeply disturbed a grown-up, let alone a child. My brother has a memory that I do not, of holding me while I screamed to see our mother in an intense state of distress and disintegration. I still carry a physical sense of my small hands balled feebly into fists and the weakness of a nine-year-old girl who wants to help, but can't. When I brought coffee and toast to her bedside, I never knew what to say and felt ashamed of my dumbness. The summer we had to leave her at home while we visited family in France, I would stare for a long time at the blue horizon and think about being with her, feeling thin and flat as an endless ocean.

On a surface level, I thought, the meaning of this psilocybin trip was straightforward: a confrontation with the fear, rage, and anguish that I'd buried a couple of decades ago because it had been too overwhelming at the time. It seemed that the mysterious physical sensation in my chest was a portal which, once opened, had flooded my body with repressed pain. My OCD, by preoccupying me with unsolvable riddles, had tried to keep me from opening the portal. The desolation of that embodied, cosmic image of losing Mom had, in its shocking awe, blown the mental illness paradigm out of the water for me. It was clear that none of this had anything to do with symptoms of illness.

I shook my head and laughed. Any pop psychologist could point out that this fear of abandonment was the unseen puppeteer in the repetitive relationship dramas of my life (I will abandon you before you have the chance to abandon me). On the surface it was so obvious, a neat line of cause and effect, packaged up in a series of hallucinogenic archetypes: the womb-like glow of love, the storm in the sky. But if the trip – with its expansiveness that I couldn't grasp, its fractal patterns whose edges I couldn't see, its bending of time and reality – had offered any immediate lesson, it's that the line between cause and effect is never neat, and the first answer you arrive at is always part of a much bigger picture.

Mom's depression cannot be decontextualised from my father's redundancy, which cannot be decontextualised from the Thatcherite privatisations in the Midlands, which destroyed livelihoods, broke up communities and cut funding to schools, schools where kids with learning difficulties were branded 'oppositional' and put on medication, like my brother had been. This tangle of social and policy issues is inseparable from the sibling violence that would break out at home when my parents' backs were turned (which was often, since Mom was frequently incapacitated and Dad was busy feeding a family of six on low income and benefits). And none of this can be decontextualised from the war, imprisonment, emigration and poverty that my grandparents resiliently stared down, nor from my inscrutably complex mix of personality traits and biology, which itself is a co-evolving story with everything around me.

I knew that it was less than ideal that I had come here to Amsterdam alone and that I didn't have the context of someone's arms to place all of this in. I called up my brother for a long chat, and that helped. As I tried to describe what it felt like to watch my love disappear into a black hole in the sky, I encountered the same dumb ineffability I'd felt back in California. When it came to altered states of consciousness, words didn't seem to be up to the job.

~

'What do you think it is about psychedelics that makes them so beyond words?' I asked Michael Pollan, the author of *How to Change Your Mind*, when I sat down with him for a podcast a few months later in 2019.

Michael: It's often been said that all mystical experiences are ineffable. William James, the great American psychologist made that point. You definitely have this feeling that you've experienced something that is beyond the reach of language

. . . As [psychedelics researcher] Bill Richards said, imagine a caveman transported to London in 2019. And he sees the Tube. And he sees aeroplanes overhead, and he sees people talking to these boxes on the side of their face. And he comes back to the cave. How does he describe it? It was big, it was loud, it was weird. He doesn't have the words for it. He doesn't have enough colours in the box of crayons to convey an experience that so few people have had . . . I was very challenged by figuring out a way to describe my own journeys without sounding like an idiot . . . You have these profound insights that are at the same time incredibly banal. You know, the classic psychedelic insight on LSD is that love is the most important thing in the universe.

Rose: Everything's connected.

Michael: Everything's connected, right? These are plati-tudes. And they're also true. So how do you get that across? We have so much protective irony around us . . . I think we defend ourselves against strong obvious feelings, or our ego does. For me, the way to write about it was to be very candid about the problem and turn to the reader at various points and say, 'Look, I know this sounds like a cliché, but think about it, what is a cliché? Where do they come from? Isn't a platitude just a truth that's been drained of emotion by repetition?' I decided I would break the fourth wall and explain to my reader when I got to a point in the narrative that either sounded too obvious or insane. Because I'm not just writing for psychonauts. To the contrary, I'm really trying to write for people who've never had this experience and give them some vicarious sense of what it is like.

Rose: You make yourself vulnerable when you're trying to write, in a similar way that you make yourself vulnerable when you're taking psychedelics?

Michael: Exactly. It's very similar, and if you're too concerned with self-protection or looking cool, forget it . . . If you're not honest with yourself, if you're not willing to share emotion, it's gonna be postured, it's not going to be authentic. It ended up being the most fun I've ever had as a writer . . .

Rose: Were there moments of discomfort though, before you reached that point of liberation? Did you cringe?

Michael: Oh yeah. I was cringing. During the trips, I'd think about things, like the importance of love and how I'm not paying enough attention to love. Afterwards I'd write it down and be like, 'ewww'. But I decided to do it anyway and actually talk about the cringe feeling. And I think that worked. Readers have to judge, but it worked for me.

Rose: I did a guided psilocybin experience recently, and I've been quite cautious not to narrativise it too quickly. Because every time I tell the story of what happened—

Michael: It changes.

Rose: Yeah, I get further away from it. In the immediate aftermath [of the trip], when I was still very fuzzy and coming down, I wrote this phrase, which at the time felt so profound and full of meaning. And I thought, this is going to be a beacon throughout my life. I'm going to return to this phrase. I read it back two days later: 'If I can do that, I can do anything.' It may as well have been a fridge magnet. But in the moment, it felt so real.

Michael: Yeah, I get it. You felt empowered. You'd done this risky thing . . . There's a famous story, it turns out to be slightly apocryphal, of William James having a big experience on nitrous oxide. He realised the secret of the universe in the middle of his trip and wrote it down. He looked at it the next morning and it said, 'The smell of fried onions.'

Rose: [*Laughs*] In the West, we have a sort of squeamishness about mysticism and spirituality—

Michael: And more in England, by the way.

Rose: Oh really? More than in the US?

Michael: At least among the psychedelic researchers – an interesting phenomenon I noticed is that in America, the researchers often talk about a high dose, complete experience as involving a 'mystical experience', or sometimes 'a mystical-type experience'. And I find the English researchers are a little allergic to that phrase. They'll talk about 'ego dissolution' as the peak of the experience . . . They're scientists, and they just don't like that tinge of spirituality, even though it is a spiritual experience. They're just different vocabularies for the same phenomenon.

Rose: For anyone that might not know, what do you mean when you say 'ego dissolution'?

Michael: Ego dissolution is the sensation many people have on a high-dose trip, when they feel safe enough to really let go – you really have to surrender to this. It's the sense that your self no longer exists, this voice in your head, this thing you identify with as you, this 'I'. I had an experience of watching it dissolve. Actually, in my case, it kind of burst into confetti, little Post-it notes. I knew that was 'me' and that I had just been exploded, detonated. And then I looked out again – and I know I'm using the 'I' now as the observer, and that's definitely a weird, paradoxical thing – I saw myself, recognisable as me, just spread out on the ground like a coat of paint. The perspective from which I was observing the scene was not myself, it wasn't my usual self, and it was completely untroubled by what I was witnessing. To this day, I don't know who that was.

Rose: It kind of sounds quite horrific. Like something out of *Terminator*.

Michael: Yeah, it should be. It's a death, you know? But it didn't feel bad, I was totally fine with it, I was reconciled. And it ended up being quite ecstatic . . . according to Freud, [the ego] defends us, it is our drive, it has a lot of adaptive value, it gets things done, it evolved for a reason. But it also is that voice in your head that's telling you you did wrong, or you could do better. Or it's the ruminating voice; it's the worrying voice. And it can torment us. I think in people who are depressed or anxious, it does torment them. So when you see it dissolve, and you don't die, you realise, 'Oh, I'm not identical to that voice. I don't have to listen to it. It's not me,' or 'It's not all of me, it's only part of me.' It's one figure in this drama of everything that's going on in your head. And that's kind of liberating. For me, that was a big takeaway of psychedelics. And it appears to be for a lot of the patients who are being treated: to escape the tyranny of the ego, even for a short period of time, opens up possibilities, new belief systems. They're not as confined by their beliefs as they were before.

Rose: Wrapped up in the psychedelics conversation is a resurgence of some older ideas in psychology, which Western medicine kind of turned its back on, like the ego and the unconscious . . . Anything resembling depth psychology is something that I was schooled to be a bit suspicious of. But I think it's really interesting now that the sciences are starting to back [these ideas] up.

Michael: It's very interesting watching the return of the unconscious. Think about behavioural economics, they're constantly talking about these unconscious biases we have, right? And if you ask them, 'Well, are you talking about an unconscious?' they really don't want to go there . . . I think psychedelics have helped it come back . . . It's often said that in the early days of psychology, Freud and Jung were brainless, they were all about the mind. And then the pendulum swung way over the other way with behaviourism. And that was mindless, it was all about the brain. And neither is right. These two things are inextricable. But we've tried to extricate them . . . That's reductive science. It tries to simplify things . . . Obviously [with psychedelics] there's a brain effect going on, and we see it, we see it on fMRI. But the mind effect appears to be what changes people. You're administering not just a drug, not just a chemical, but an *experience* to people. And it's only when they have that experience – call it ego dissolution, mystical experience – that they change. That's a weird model, but it makes sense. If you think about trauma . . . there is a life experience that changes the brain and changes people's minds as well, in a profound way, a negative way. Is it possible that a very positive and equally disruptive experience could change the mind in a positive direction?

Rose: What I think is quite enjoyable about the psychedelics conversation is that it reintroduces some of the poetry of those older psychoanalysts back into the conversation on mental health, like Jung especially, and Freud. These guys were amazing writers. When I was trying to conceptualise my psychedelic experience on magic truffles, I hadn't really been able to articulate it until I came across something that Jung wrote about 'the night sea journey'. He conceptualised going into the subconscious as this journey on a boat in a storm in the night.[2] I feel like modern psychiatric literature abandoned [this kind of poetry].

Michael: Yeah, we're back in the world of symbols and archetypes, and the fact is, as uncomfortable as this makes some neuroscientists feel, you can't penetrate consciousness without talking about experience, phenomenology and what not. What is the lived experience? You correlate that with brain states, fine, but storytelling is essential if you're trying to capture consciousness.

Rose: Was it your 5-MeO-DMT experience that was a real horror show?
[*5-MeO-DMT is a tryptamine psychedelic found in many plant species and in the glandular secretions of a species of toad.*]

Michael: It's funny, I often ask audiences, when I decide I'm going to read a little passage, 'Do you want to hear a good or a bad trip?' They always say, 'Bad trip.' It's universal. People want to know, 'What's the worst case before I think about doing this?' So for me, it was 5-MeO-DMT. This is the smoked venom of the Sonoran Desert toad. The venom by itself is toxic, but you can smoke it. No toads are harmed in the harvesting process, basically you gently milk the toads' glands . . .

Rose: This is beside the point, but are they farmed, or . . . ?

Michael: [*Laughs*] No. We haven't gotten to that point. These are wild toads. So after hemming and hawing and going back and forth, and my ego saying, 'Don't do that,' I decided I would do it. And it was pretty horrifying. You take one puff, on this vape situation, and then even before you exhale, you're just gone. You fall back, there's no onset, you feel like you've been strapped to the outside of a rocket that is rising and shuddering and going faster and faster and breaking through clouds and trying to get up into space, and you feel the G-force pulling down on your face. And your sense of self is instantly exploded. Then everything else goes too: matter, time, everything is a storm of what felt like pure energy that was in my skull but extended outside of it also . . . I had my mantra of 'trust, surrender. Trust, surrender'. And I kept trying to say it, but it was useless. I couldn't think. It was too chaotic to have thoughts. It was terrifying. I thought, 'Oh my god, this is death, or this is the passage to death because nothing exists any more.'

The best thing about it, is it only lasts about ten minutes. It felt like an eternity. But at a certain point, I started coming down, and I realised, 'Wow, that's the same song I heard when I lay down.' And then I very quickly felt reality reassemble. And it was ecstatic actually. This was the payoff: that I was still alive . . . I was lying down and I had a blanket over me, and I reached down and felt my thighs. *Oh, I have a body . . . You exist, I exist.* And not only that, I felt the Earth. The floor. I felt time passing as I listened to this music. And I had the most profound sense of gratitude I've ever had, not just for being alive, which most of us have felt at some point, but that there is anything and not nothing.[3]

Steelworker

The Cartwrights were
labourers and chain
makers in England's
Black Country. Great
Uncle Harry, a bin man
who lived in a caravan at
the tip, had received the
last recorded flogging at
the local workhouse. I
don't know what he'd
done, but I like the idea
of a rogue in the family.
His brother, my grandad
George, was conscripted
from his steelworker job
into the British Navy
during the Second World
War, where he saw a ship
carrying a thousand men
get struck by German
bombers and explode.
When his fleet landed
in New York, he met
and fell in love with
Catherine, a devout
Catholic who'd emigrated
from a poverty-stricken
Scotland and was
working as a maid for
the mayor of New York.
George took Catherine
back to England's coal-
black heart, where they
married and tried for a
baby, but could
not conceive.

Connective tissue

'Relationships are the crucible in which our lives unfold as they shape our life story, molding our identity and giving birth to the experience of who we are, and liberating – or constraining – who we can become . . . the stories that bind us to each other . . . [are] located deeply in a between-domain of our relational lives.'[1]

Professor Daniel Siegel, psychiatrist

I always thought I knew what trauma was. I'd learned about shellshock in school, about soldiers returning from the First World War with mystifying symptoms. Some shivered, some panicked, some writhed against terrors no one else could see. Most couldn't sleep or slept too much. Some banged their fists against their ears, terrified by sudden sounds. Some were numb and mute. Some, with their boots still caked in muck from the trenches where they'd fired mortars or gone over the top, cried out in the night for their mothers. Aggressive outbursts, nightmares and intrusive memories of battle were common.

The doctors at the time had theories about what was wrong with these men: perhaps they'd been poisoned by carbon monoxide, or they had cerebral lesions caused by falling shells. But modern doctors debunked these old ideas, discovering that these soldiers had a mental illness which would come to be called post-traumatic stress disorder, PTSD. (We tend to associate the creation of a psychiatric diagnostic category and its inclusion in diagnostic manuals as progress, just like we tend to assume that receiving a diagnosis will lead to getting targeted help for that problem. And yet, while outcomes have dramatically improved in many other corners of medicine, mainstream psychiatry continues to fail to offer a reliable treatment for PTSD.)

As I got older, I came to understand that trauma wasn't just about veterans. PTSD could happen to anyone who'd survived acute, catastrophic and out-of-the-ordinary experiences. Survivors of house fires, car crashes, violent and sexual assaults, near-drownings, freak accidents, botched anaesthetics, and natural disasters. Those who've witnessed the mass-scale devastation of pillage, displacement of populations and genocide.

We've met these people in films many times. The constraints of film as a visual medium have created a skewed impression of the phenomenology of their suffering. Their behaviour has to play well on screen, it has to be dramatic. Explosive anger plays better than seamlessly repressed anger; photorealistic flashbacks play better than vague ineffable pain; rocking back and forth plays better than endless numbness. Sudden breakdowns play better than years and years of high-functioning survival. Clear causality plays better than muddy uncertainty. You'll often see a trauma story unfold over a series of flashbacks, each informing your understanding of the present action and adding to a breadcrumb trail that leads to a climactic and usually simplistic revelation.

Partial representations like this are one reason why I never assumed that someone like me, with my loving family and my ordinary life, could be traumatised. Real trauma can be much more complex and harder to identify.

~

Humans are extremely resilient and adaptive animals. When we face a situation that our systems perceive as a threat, our bodies get ready to take self-protective action of some kind. We might get tense, anxious and ready for conflict. Or we may shut down and disengage. Usually, the threat passes and we're able to realign. The physiological 'charge' of stress, the readiness for threat, is discharged, and the cognitive parts of your brain process all this into narrative – something happened, it's not happening any more. There is a sense of completion as the event is metabolised and consigned to memory. We do this to a lesser or greater extent every day. We're good at it.

But according to trauma theory, if the threat is over-whelming, the system ceases to be able to complete a healthy stress response. To protect you from the resulting firestorm of unmanageable stress, the system brings out a last line of defence: the trauma response. It pours suppressant foam all over the flames, scoops up the wreckage, puts it in landfill and buries it, far enough away from you that you can at least survive. Into the depths along with it are tipped any emotions and sensations associated with the original threat that were too big for you to bear in the moment. But the burial is not perfect. It is a crude and messy job and involves a huge amount of energy. Your system can, at great exhaustive effort, suppress feelings, but it cannot forget them entirely. Fragments remain on the surface. We spend our lives pawing through them trying to make sense of ourselves, having no idea that most of the puzzle is deep down inside us.

Because all of this is a subconscious mechanism, in that you didn't choose it and weren't aware of it, your thinking brain was never able to make sense of the traumatic event, to create clear memories out of it, put words to it or archive it. There is no completion, no sense of an ending. Under ordinary circumstances, the brain is an excellent storyteller; it is constantly rescripting the self to make meaning out of the twists and turns of life and slot them into a coherent schema about who we are. Many people with trauma seem to have partially lost the sense data that would help order their experiences and give them satisfying meaning. So we feel stuck in a never-ending story of maddeningly repeating beats. We meet new characters, move to new locations, play new roles. But our ancient survival system is denying us access to the only ending the cognitive mind cares about: 'I'm safe now.'

In his book, *Slaughterhouse-Five*, writer Kurt Vonnegut layers images and emotions in a non-linear structure. It impacted me deeply when I read it as a teenager, before I understood that what was being described were traumatic flashbacks. One day, the lead character, Billy Pilgrim, feels like he's having a heart attack when he sees a barbershop quartet perform. 'He could find no explanation for why the song had affected him so grotesquely,' Vonnegut writes, 'here was proof that he had a great big secret somewhere inside, and he could not imagine what it was.'[2] Soon, the reader gets an insight when we are shown the moment from Billy's past when he saw four soldiers standing in the rubble after the bombing of Dresden. When Billy is sickened and confused by the barbershop quartet, he is looking through what Vonnegut brilliantly calls a 'time window'[3], feeling the interminable emotions that stretch between this dimension and that one.

It's easy to imagine how an overwhelming experience like the bombing of a city, or those listed above (natural disaster, assault, etc.) could trigger this kind of trauma response and lead to psychological fragmentation, but it can also arise from less acute but still very serious forms of adversity. These include, but are not limited to, food and housing insecurity; excessive use of alcohol or drugs in the home; discrimination based on race, sexual orientation or class; the ongoing mental distress of a family member; physical disability of a family member; and witnessing violence.

Trauma not only potentially results from bad things happening, but also from the absence of good things happening. Many kinds of absence can be traumatising and leave us with a sense of void throughout our lives: lack of employment, lack of purpose; and lack of connection to nature. Sometimes the lack is so total and historic we don't even think of it as a problem, even if it's affecting us on a deep level. I was stopped in my tracks when I read how psychiatrist Bruce D. Perry describes the West's loss of community as 'relational poverty'.[4] We are relationally impoverished, atomised into small, productive family units with decreasing interdependence between them, increased emphasis on the primacy of romantic relationships, little intergenerational knowledge-sharing, almost no serendipitous interaction (message before you call; call before you pop in) and fewer and fewer communal rites.

In childhood, loss can be experienced through the physical absence of a caregiver (a successful banker who works all hours may be able to provide material luxury, but be unable to provide the regular cuddles and reassurances their child needs); or the emotional absence of a caregiver, sometimes called proximate separation (a stay-at-home parent may be physically present all day but, because of their own unresolved emotional difficulties, unable to engage in the physical play their child needs).

In 1975, the first Still Face Experiment was conducted. A mother and baby sat opposite each other. The mother, who was usually responsive and attuned to her child, was instructed to suddenly adopt a blank expression. Researchers recorded how the baby responded. At first, the baby tried to interact with the mother to elicit a reaction in ways it knew how: smiling, pointing, grabbing. After a couple of minutes of being met with the blank face, the baby withdrew, angled themselves away and grew overwhelmed with hopelessness.[5] This is one of the most replicated findings in childhood development.[6] It suggests that something as seemingly subtle as not receiving reciprocal interactions with a caregiver can have a profound negative impact on wellbeing.

Whether through the presence of bad or the absence of good, if a child's environment is chronically stressful, they can start to feel alone in emotions that they do not understand and cannot express. Perhaps because expressing themselves would inflame their environmental stressors further. Anger cannot be discharged through shouts and tantrums if you risk provoking someone. Fear cannot be discharged through sprinting legs if you've never been outside on your own before. Longing cannot be articulated if that's all you know. Since a child's life is dependent on the stability of its environment and primary caregivers, anything that threatens that stability can feel like a threat to life. If a child can't change the stressors in their environment (when can they ever?), they're likely to believe that the problem lies in them (*I'm unlovable, I'm worthless, I deserve this*). The alternative is understanding that the problem is 'out there' in the world, and because this idea is synonymous with not being safe, it is too terrible to contemplate. 'Trauma hijacks our stories,'[7] as psychiatrist Dr Paul Conti put it succinctly, and can show up as shame, hypersensitivity, numbness, aggression, passivity, addiction, aversion to intimacy, insomnia and a broad range of other feelings and behaviours.

But we should also be cautious about broadening the definition of trauma. Professor Nick Haslam coined the phrase 'concept creep' in reference to the 'semantic inflation' that happens when definitions of harm are gradually expanded.[8] For example, how the definition of addiction has expanded from substance addiction to include other kinds of repetitive compulsive behaviour like sex addiction or work addiction; or how the definition of bullying, which in the 1970s referred almost exclusively to school-yard aggression, now encompasses adult interactions in the workplace and remote cyber bullying. Indeed, how the concept of trauma has expanded to include things like collective trauma and vicarious trauma. Haslam says that concept creep has had ambivalent consequences. While it's been positive in shedding light on previously overlooked forms of harm, it has also diffused our warranted focus on some of the worst forms of it.

I share his ambivalence, especially now that social media and alternative healing, and the saccharine place where those two things meet, has become saturated with trauma language. Where exposure to divergent political views is equated to exposure to violence; where important psychological skills like 'boundary setting' and 'cocooning' are used to justify the selfishness and flakiness that are making our lives worse; where people routinely use words like 'triggered' and 'harmed' in place of 'upset' or 'annoyed'. But who's to judge?

Sometimes I find myself stifling an eyeroll when peers who seem to have had relatively stress-free lives describe themselves as having trauma, though that's hardly fair. I'm not in their head and I don't know what it's like to be them, and policing language leads to nowhere good. Attempts to control the words that others use to express their inner life are almost always part of a divisive, possessive narrative, itself a product of pain: 'You don't know what it's like to be me.' The traumatised and the not-traumatised, the diagnosed and the undiagnosed, the ill and the well. There are no clear demarcations between us. We are not at odds with each other.

Trauma is a diffuse construct, in that people with trauma are not a homogenous category. While adverse experiences can leave imprints on the body and brain that are comparable to physical injuries, and childhood abuse has been shown to cause neurological changes in victims,[9] trauma is not currently diagnosable with objective tests. While we can learn from what medicalisation has achieved with its PTSD label (the recognition of severe trauma as incredibly serious), I don't think we should outsource the authority to arbitrate who does and doesn't have trauma to medical professionals. We can foster an exceptionalism around the half-living, half-dead nightmare of trauma at its most debilitating without ring-fencing it as illness or pretending that anyone knows where to draw the lines on the spectrum.

~

Though I was in a state of self-protective denial, I had always known what I'd been through as a child. Specific visual memories are few and far between, but I have always remembered, in broad strokes at least, the bad stuff that happened. It's become popular in psychedelic healing circles for people to approach trips on the hunt for repressed memories, but I was very cautious not to do that, and no new autobiographical facts ever emerged from my trips.

I did however retrieve emotional data (pain, love, fear, anger), which seemed to have been lost in time. A kind of 'body knowledge' that had been marooned on an island that I couldn't walk to, visible in the distance but inaccessible to my grown-up thinking mind. It's like I knew about my past but also *didn't know*, at the same time. I've puzzled over this a lot. How could I know, for example, that I routinely experienced violence for many years, if I only have a couple of single-frame visual memories? I've come to understand that my memories were not lost exactly, but disintegrated. Holistic memory involves the integration of logical, fact-based information, and contextual, emotional and somatic information.

Clinical psychologist Frank Tallis offers this theory of the brain activity associated with trauma:

> Sensory information passes through a structure in the brain called the thalamus, where data streams are integrated so that memories can be retrieved holistically . . . But when we are overwhelmed by a traumatic experience, the thalamus stops synthesising data streams. Information can only be stored in a fragmentary form. Memories of the trauma are inaccessible or discontinuous. There is no logical sequence of events to remember, only islands of sensation and emotion. The left hemisphere of the brain is deactivated, and experience cannot be understood as a series of causes and effects. The story we tell ourselves about ourselves becomes confused and breaks down.[10]

This description reminds me of something we talk about in screenwriting: connective tissue – i.e. the logical flow that gets the plot from A to B convincingly. Sometimes, when you start editing material and something feels off, the problem can be a lack of connective tissue enabling the audience to join the dots and stay orientated. But the absence can be quite subtle. A void is more difficult to identify and remedy than a glaring error.

There's a running joke on film sets when something is going wrong: 'Fix it in post.' It means fix it in post-production – i.e.

let the editor sort this mess out. It's usually used sardonically when something clearly cannot be fixed in post and you know that you're handing a bag of shite over to the editor. Actors can't act? Fix it in post. Scene out of focus? Fix it in post.

The editor is the goalkeeper in filmmaking, the last line of defence, often the hero. I like to think of my own little inner editor, sat at her desk in the 1990s, assessing the incoming material, feeling overwhelmed, and thinking, 'What the fuck am I going to do with all this?' All this emotion, sensation and cognition, too voluminous to label or place in order. Like all good editors, she works magic to cut things out and piece things together, but she knows that the connective tissue is weak and that the story doesn't make sense. In the main, coherency and emotional depth are sacrificed; key visuals and audio are lost. She packages up the edit, sends it off and crosses her fingers: 'This is far from perfect but it's the best that I can do.' After a quarter of a century, with the help of some powerful psychedelics, I finally retrieved some of the missing emotional beats and got my story flowing again.

But even this reading of what trauma is and how psychedelics work, and the neatness of the metaphors I've used to bring it alive, should not be gripped with any force. There is an inclination, especially now that concepts of trauma have exploded into popular awareness, to overlay meaning too quickly and literally on to altered states of consciousness. It's true that the sudden bolt of realisation I had in the wake of my big trip in Amsterdam – that my distress stems from repressed traumatic pain – has remained stable over several years. So too have my insights about the circumstances that led to that pain. It all feels as powerfully and ineffably true now as it did then. But there's an uncomfortable possibility I still keep on the table: if you spend a couple of years drenching yourself in trauma culture, as I had done by 2019, then go into a psychedelic trip expecting to meet your trauma, the expectation can influence the content that comes up.

In 2023, I spoke to the University of Auckland's Dr Tehseen Noorani, a social scientist and the co-founder of experimental think tank, Lentil Lab. Tehseen coined the phrase 'the Pollan Effect', to describe the impact that Michael Pollan's *How to Change Your Mind*, has had on clinical trial participants' expectations of psychedelic experiences, and how these priors might be influencing trial results.

Rose: Lots of Westerners are undergoing psychedelic experiences expecting to meet their trauma, then coming out feeling like they have. And this is weird territory, but to what extent do you think that is really happening? Or is this traumatic content shaped by their expectations?

Tehseen: To an extent, I do think people are having healing psychedelic experiences. These might be super amped by their expectation that they're going to heal. But it's interesting to analyse what happens when things don't go according to plan, and these experiences don't follow that same mastery narrative of getting exactly what you want. People can get huge disappointment effects that can be devastating, especially if people think this is some kind of last-shot miracle cure for treatment-resistant depression or whatever, and then it doesn't go as they'd hoped. But yes, I think on average, psychedelics are having larger healing effects because of enhanced placebo through expectancy.

Rose: To play devil's advocate and counter that slightly (and this is a phenomenological point so I certainly won't hang my hat on it), psychedelics do seem to take you to a place beyond where expectation can reach. At least that's what it feels like. You often find yourself in these regressed states, re-experiencing babyhood or whatever, and that baby has no idea who Michael Pollan is. It's difficult to unpack because what the hell do we know? That regression experience itself could also be a projection of the infantilising psychothera-peutic culture we live in. But my sense is that at some point, if you go deep enough into these experiences, the ability of culture and expectation to shape the content is left at the door.

Tehseen: That's certainly possible. So without wanting to counter it head on, there are a few other ways to approach this. Think about the course of a ship – change the course just a tiny amount, you won't see the effects straight away, but over great distances, it will end up in a very different place because of that tiny adjustment . . . The relationship between expectation and outcome is not necessarily linear. Where we end up could seem unrelated to our expectations, and yet there might be a path of dependency that's very hard to trace. This is why we need to think carefully about practices of preparation and integration. There's a hegemonic view in therapy culture, where we expect to be given lots of truths about ourselves. For me, it's more a question of, what's the most fruitful avenue for an individual and the most capacious interpretive lens for them?

Rose: I think for anyone going into these psychedelic experiences, a neutral framing might be helpful, whereby we hold insights lightly. We can search for meaning and use it to the extent to which it's useful. But also be prepared to let it go.[11]

In short, I can't be certain that the 'trauma work' I've done while tripping is not merely a projection of an internalised zeitgeist. Crucially, I don't need to be certain. Perhaps the single most important skill that mental health sufferers can learn is to hold cherished stories, models, and insights lightly and to go into 'healing' experiences, as far as possible, with what Zen Buddhists call *shoshin* – beginner's mind. If you have a beginner's mind, you try to let go of preconceptions, foster an attitude of openness and are willing to be surprised. (Psychotherapy can sometimes run counter to that goal if you're encouraged to frame your experiences according to whichever therapeutic tradition your therapist has trained in.)

Buddhist monks ritualise *shoshin* by spending many painstaking days creating fantastically intricate images of mandalas out of coloured sand, only to ceremonially sweep the sand away and destroy their own work. The practice reminds them of the certainty of impermanence and the futility of clinging to any one moment. By trying to cultivate *shoshin*, we can help to inoculate ourselves against overinterpreting the meaning of thoughts and feelings. I had this modelled to me on a meditation retreat by my exceptionally wise Buddhist teacher, Kirsten Kratz.

'I have this lump in my throat that won't go away,' a fellow meditator asked her. 'I keep asking myself, what does it mean? What's it trying to say?'

Kirsten paused. Then replied, 'What's it trying to say when it's not there?'

~

I have spent a lot of time at psychedelics parties and conferences, meeting people who've made healing their identity, who are compelled to keep psychedelically turning themselves inside out, certain that the answer about how to live would eventually shake loose. These are the trauma chasers, the tornado hunters, who risk destroying themselves in the search for the next big one. If you get channelled into meeting like-minded people and consuming like-minded messages, it's easy to get swept up in this vortical energy; no one is impervious to it. I certainly wasn't. I had to learn to recognise when my trauma hunt itself was becoming a kind of psychological 'look over there', enabling me to ignore the systemic conditions of modern life that were draining me: consumerism, isolation from community, the forty-hour work week.

As the psychedelic renaissance gathers pace, two possibilities can check and balance each other, and maybe enrich each other. Yes, the West's current obsession with trauma is probably leading more people to narrowly identify with trauma and therefore overlook other helpful interpretations. By holding a magnifying glass over isolated interpersonal traumas, psychedelic culture can repeat the reductionism of the biomedical model by ignoring our broader relationship to everything around us. Also, yes: trauma is as real and true as grief, and psychedelics seem to be excellent tools for exploring the pain (and joy) of the past.

I wrote about my happy memories in *Pure*, of which there are many. I was immensely privileged in lots of ways. Our house was full of books, animals and birds, and we spent time in nature every week. Every night he could, Dad read us stories, never too tired to do the silly voices which made each character come alive. My whole head fit on his shoulder, my brother's on his other. His voice buzzed through his chest as he read us *Asterix* or *Old Bear*. Playtime was creative and adventurous and messy (raw jelly cubes stick to wallpaper if you throw hard enough; hardened dog shit is an excellent missile). Many of our family friends were eccentrics and outsiders. The door often knocked with drop-ins. The belly laughter of people who'd had rough lives regularly raised the roof.

When I wrote about these memories, I was not consciously leaving anything out, or deliberately painting a partial picture: this was the full picture as I was able to cognitively understand it. The following passage from *Pure*, written ten years before I wrote this book, is indicative of the tactical blind spot that trauma can create: 'Any hardship, [my parents] hid from me – mental illness and physical illness and benefits – as the baby I was protected from the enormity of these things. I was kept safe and happy and oblivious. So I can't say why I started faking asthma attacks when I was eight years old . . . Finding my lies rewarded with love, I'd be rushed by a fawning dinner lady to the potpourri-smelling reception area . . . Sometimes they'd let me go home and Mom would give me warm Ribena.'[12]

The clues are right there. I'm saying that my behaviour rewarded me with love, while at the same time saying that I don't know why I behaved the way I did. I'm saying I'm oblivious to my motives while stating my motives. I have come to the compassionate view that there's something elegant and tender about the mind's ability to do this – to hide in plain sight from itself. Poet David Whyte put it beautifully:

> Refusing to face what we are not yet ripe and ready to face can help us to live through the more than enough difficulties of the present . . . Denial is a beautiful transitional state every human being inhabits before they are emancipated into the next larger context and orphaned, often against their will, from their old and very familiar home . . . it is a necessary dynamic, so that the overpowering elements of a waiting, terrifying, universe can be held for now, over the horizon.[13]

I had tried to pretend with *Pure* that my problems did not involve my family. The medical paradigm facilitated this, enabling me to cast my distress as isolated from my relationships. But the cracks in the pretence had started to show. When I'd promoted the book on a BBC show called *Woman's Hour*, and the host had asked me how my family had responded to my work, I burst out crying on live radio. My heart had been sending messages that I'd been successfully stopping at the neck and shoving back down. Now, in the wake of my trip to Amsterdam, it was obvious that my mental health problems had always been inextricably tied to the adversity of my childhood. But how could I talk about that without hurting the people I love?

Altered states of consciousness can reveal to us – and I think this is one of those moments where Michael Pollan would caveat a platitude – that love is the truest story in the universe. Trauma, via societal adversities that pick at the fabric of families, dragging them into financial hardship, meaningless work and mind-numbing medication, can bomb our connecting bridges and make us defensive against pain. And therefore defensive against love in its full vulnerability. I knew I would have to find a way to have the conversations I'd been avoiding my whole life. It wouldn't be as simple as acknowledging the obvious fact that no one was to blame and that everyone had been doing their best in an immensely stressful situation. I would have to go deeper.

Matches

'She wanted to warm herself, people said.'[1]

The Little Match Girl, Hans Christian Andersen

I was 18 years old. It was my first year at university and my first year living away from home. I was in my halls of residence bedroom getting ready for a Halloween party. I was dressed as a convincing Wonder Woman, if Wonder Woman shopped down the slut aisle of Poundland. At the time I was drinking a lot and throwing up my food most days. The antidepressants that I'd been prescribed had blunted my emotions and I'd started cutting my skin to cut through the numbness.

With the heavy pre-drinking well underway, my stomach muscles tightened as I looked at my phone and saw my dad calling from his mobile, not the landline. My body had already guessed what he was about to tell me: Mom, who had been bed-bound by depression for many weeks, had been admitted to psychiatric hospital again.

The hospital was, and is, called Bushey Fields, a name presumably inspired by the surrounding industrial estates, dual carriageways, steel yards and meat wholesalers. For us it was a helpful shorthand for when someone we knew ended up in there, which happened quite often. 'So and so has gone up Bushey Fields.' Say no more. My new flatmates were not versed in the shorthand, so I had to give them the full explanation. They didn't know what to say. 'Mental hospital' is a grenade in conversation. People fret with it. Hop about with it. They look around hoping someone will have it off them.

Later that semester, a GP, Dr Harris, looked over the rim of her glasses to inspect the older cuts on my left arm. There were six deeper cuts, each about an inch long that would become scars.

'Have you self-harmed since I last saw you?' she said.

'No,' I said.

Her eyes landed on a new cut on my right arm.

'I did it by accident in the kitchen,' I said. I was telling the truth. It'd happened a couple of days before when I'd snagged it on a cupboard. I'd cursed my clumsiness. It looked deliberate and I knew that this would affect my credit rating.

The doctor angled my arm for a better look and raised her eyebrows at me. I rolled down my sleeve and shrank from her incredulous gaze. She asked me if the antidepressants had helped. I said 'no' and instantly felt that this was the wrong answer or that I should have softened it somehow. She asked me how the counselling she'd referred me to was going. I told her it was going well because I didn't want to displease her any further. I left the doctor's surgery in what

I would later recognise as a dissociative state. The world looked plasticky and unreal as I walked slowly home.

As I grew up, like all of us I would come to know people with dysfunctional lives and reflect that many of them, whether or not they had a diagnosis – ironically, some of the most dysfunctional and unhappy never identify as being ill – were struggling with iterations of the same question: why do I behave the way I behave? Why do I do the destructive things that I do? Why do I keep doing something I'm ashamed of? Why am I drinking/shagging/fighting/shirking my life away?

As for me, why was I cutting myself and throwing up my food? I'd been told that my behaviours were caused by dysfunction in my brain, a dysfunction that the drugs were designed to target. But the drugs were making me feel like I wasn't on the planet. Nothing made sense. My behaviour was a mystery to me.

This chapter is about my attempt to unravel the mystery.

~

Trace the big hairline crack across the bobbled plaster of my Amsterdam hotel room, and follow it over the North Sea seabed, up through the dense anaerobic mud of the Thames, across the earth of the city and up to the ceiling of my east London flat, underneath which I sit alone, one month after my psilocybin experience, measuring out a bomb of MDMA.

I have no way of knowing whether my Amsterdam trip would have been quite so horrific if it had been facilitated differently. I've read that traumatic 'bad trips' happen even in optimal settings, and that the 'badness' can be beneficial if it's part of a process of 'uprooting' trauma. But I didn't know if mine had been badness that leads to goodness, or badness that leads to more badness. I don't know of any official bodies I can ask; no helpline I could ring to talk about what I went through. Later, several underground psychedelic guides will tell me that the sitters should not have left me alone; that in their opinion, the salt bath decision should not have been left until I was high, especially since it involved me removing clothes; that the sitters should not have been so high themselves that they became engrossed in their own experience; and that problems generally arise when sitters impose too much of their own ego and personal taste on the experience.

My sitters were variously dancing around the room, putting on their favourite tracks, stroking each other's hands and gazing tearfully into each other's eyes. At one point during the deepest part of the trip when I was crying, Allison, presumably as part of her energy work, was dangling her hair on the skin of my arm. In such a deep state of disorientation, this felt confusing and icky to me, and had not been discussed ahead of time.

This is what the psychedelic renaissance can look like in the hands of well-meaning but naive people who fancy themselves as the next Instagram shaman or rockstar traumatologist but have no cultural inheritance or therapeutic training to guide them. Healing and spiritual practices have always attracted wannabe gurus bent on enrolling others in their healing fantasy, with all the problematic power dynamics that that entails. Trip sitting is no exception. Evangelism and cliche abound in a nascent psychedelic healer culture that creaks with growing pains and can attract people who don't have the requisite groundedness and psychological maturity to be subtly attuned to the emotions of others. Most people who want to retrain as psychedelic therapists, typically off the back of their own psychedelic experiences, probably shouldn't. I meet these people often at events, people who seriously describe themselves as 'bringers of joy' and 'sooth-sayers' and 'leaders of light'. At a friend's party in 2021, a gong-bath practitioner told me, not metaphorically, that she was part-goddess, that her alien goddess ancestors had mated with monkeys and that's why she had the healing power that she did. When I looked around and no one else was reacting, I made a mental note to spend less time in places like that. I notice that when people claim alien ancestry (it's happened since) they always think they're descended from wise, deity aliens, never boring, narcissist aliens. Same with the past-life people. Everyone always thinks they were a warrior in a past life, or a medicine woman, or an outlaw, or a *sage*. No one's past life was ever mundane, or unremarkable. Considering ego death is routinely touted as the apotheosis of the psychedelic experience, the egotism that abounds in the psychedelic world is astonishing.

In 2023, I would go to a psychedelics conference called Psych Symposium where a panel of experts comprising psychedelics researchers and clinical trial facilitators discussed psychedelic therapy. The panellists agreed that the roles of trip sitters and psychedelic therapists are not yet defined, and that aside from any label, it's a person's human qualities of humility and compassion that determine whether or not they'll be a supportive companion for your journey.

There's a gold rush in the industry, with various institutions rolling out accreditation and training programs in a race to establish the definitive psychedelic therapist qualification. I worry that this rush is serving professionals' career goals more than it is serving patients' personal goals. Panellist Nadav Liam Modlin, the psychedelic therapy lead at King's College London, said that at this early stage in the renaissance, it's the patients who should be training guides – we need to be listened to carefully and the qualities we say we're looking for in a guide are what matter most.[2]

What I look for in a guide is a serious person who is warm, smart, curious, and humble, who is deeply established and at ease in their own life and body. Someone discerning, who's probably been around a while, not a trying-to-be-influencer who trip-sits to supplement their essential oils pyramid-scheme income. I'm sceptical of any self-billed healer who uses capital letters as a sales technique. 'You could CHANGE your life TODAY.' Stay back, troll! Or any guide who talks about their own transformation ad nauseum. For me, a trip sitter is a trusted friend and mentor who is respectful of boundaries yet physically affectionate; who can get enough of their own ego out of the room to generously facilitate the unfolding of a process in me. As the brilliant underground mushroom guide I would eventually find in the UK told me, it's an act of service. If you're looking for your God-is-a-DJ moment, maybe just host a party instead? You'd probably help more people.

When asked on the conference panel what he thought makes a good psychedelic therapist, Modlin said, 'There are lots of ways to answer that question. The most dramatic version is that your psychedelic guide should be a person you'd want by your side when you're dying.'[3]

I later interviewed the panel chair, psychoanalytic psychotherapist, Timmy Davis, who's been a therapist in the room during psychedelic clinical trials and is the policy director of the Psilocybin Access Rights campaign.

'The history of therapy is marginalised people not getting access to this quite middle-class pursuit,' I said to Davis. 'Is psychedelic therapy always something that an individual does with a therapist or two, or can we open-source the knowledge about how to do this stuff safely in community settings?'

'My organising principle around this is "let a thousand flowers bloom",' Davis said. 'The point of regulation and governance is to keep people safe and reduce risks. I think there should be a route to get professional mental health treatment in a societally sanctioned way, for the people that want it. There should be another route where people can do it in whatever way they want as sovereign adults, which is controversial.'

'Take skydiving,' Davis said. 'The first couple of times you jump out of a plane, you are strapped to the body of someone who's done it several times. And then slowly you learn how to dive in different ways. With psychedelics, an apprenticeship model could work, when you have an initiation in a medical setting, and are free to move out and experiment, but essentially always free to move back into a more controlled, held environment.'[4]

~

Back in 2019, I can't even dream of such a supportive model. All I can do is speculate that my psyche didn't feel safe enough in Amsterdam to surrender and so I was abruptly sucked out of the most frightening part of the trip. For certain, I am now terrified of psilocybin and of trip sitters.

My mystical experience in 2017 had suggested to me that my thoughts were a barrier of some kind. My aching chest gave me a lantern to follow to the foot of that barrier that my psilocybin trip then cracked open, briefly illuminating what my thoughts had been trying to hold back. But a glimpse wasn't enough. I want to know more about the side of my psyche that I saw that day. I am more desperate than ever to hack my brain and heal.

Without realising, I am falling for the biggest canard of the psychedelic renaissance: that psychedelics alone can cure you like pills that you pop. Now, a month after Amsterdam, finding myself not only not cured but actually more anxious and more wary of trusting strangers, I feel the way that psychiatric treatments have always made me feel: an incurable failure. Meanwhile, as usual, I cannot see the void: the ways in which my life lacks the community support and embodied practices that might have bedded any healing insights in.

I'm on the waitlists for as many clinical psychedelics trials as I think I reasonably qualify for, but I've heard nothing back. So I'm going it alone. Having followed the clinical trials of MDMA for a couple of years, I have decided to pivot to a different drug. The Multidisciplinary Association for Psychedelic Studies (MAPS) has conducted studies which they say prove that MDMA, in combination with psychedelic therapy, massively reduces the symptoms of post-traumatic stress disorder, a diagnosis I now feel more closely aligned to than OCD. But MDMA therapy won't be legal in the UK for years, which means that, for now, we can look but we can't touch. I know that on my own I can't recreate the relational element of MDMA therapy, which they say is so crucial. But what am I supposed to do, live another half-decade in hell? I can't wait patiently any more. I've been a patient too long.

Apparently, mindset and setting are as important with MDMA as with psilocybin. I've muted the doorbell. My phone is off. I have an eye mask, and an array of soft duvets and pillows on my bed that I have spritzed with lavender. I have an electronic playlist playing. From where I lie on the bed I can see my favourite tree out the window, and I have my notepad in front of me.

At 2.30 p.m., after weighing out a standard trial dose on micro scales, I take the first bomb. When I feel the first *whomp* in my chest, I stand up and start taking a wash off the drying rack. The washing smells like the laundry cupboard in my old house and feels fluffy against my hands, and with another *whomp* I start to melt into a diffuse feeling of glowing softness. I take an armful of washing and press my face into it. Whites and pinks shimmer in my vision as I sigh into the bundle. This is the most singularly exquisite thing I've ever experienced. I am back beyond the veil, with no intrusive thoughts, and no knowledge of them ever having existed. I let out big blissful sighs at the reminder that this place is accessible. An hour in, I lie down and put on an eye mask. Occasionally I surface and write notes in handwriting so loose it's almost illegible. I barely write in prose. Just a series of statements, as each wave of the trip rolls through:

This is your home.
I have resources.
I am surrounded by people who love me.

You can't deny it hurts.
Your capacity for love is immense.
I have agency.
Wrapped in love.

How do I return?
I'm returning home.
Home is within me.

Maybe it's still too painful for you to inhabit these memories.
But it won't always be.
Everything in time.

My body is turned into a living metaphor: it has become my home. My small physical frame has become a large shelter in which my life can be housed. The past has become a place that can be safely visited when I'm ready – a literal space to be explored with touch.

I remove my eye mask and take in my surroundings. The crack on the ceiling, which hasn't bothered me for the last five hours, starts to bother me again, and with a soft pang of grief I realise that the trip is ending. I stay lying down, looking at the tree, for an hour.

The experience had surpassed any expectations of depth, intensity and strangeness. I am dumbfounded and fascinated. What is a drug like this going to do to our mental health system? Surely it will redefine what therapy can mean, and therefore rock the mental health industry to the core?

~

I explored MDMA's potential over the next two years through many more solo journeys. What struck me during those trips is the way that MDMA seems to turn psychological theories into embodied experiences. Ideas that had always failed to cut through with psychotherapy (like 'face your fear', 'you're not alone', 'what you resist, persists') become literally tangible on MDMA as the drug somehow uses the body as a medium to make you *feel*, not just understand. MDMA is sometimes called an *entactogen*, from Greek and Latin roots meaning 'touching within'.

After a decade and a half of failed talk therapy, it was a huge relief in 2019 finally to be in touch with my feelings rather than talking endlessly about them; to be feeling my way through my problems rather than trying to think myself out of them. 'Unlike thinking', writes Buddhist teacher, Stephan Bodian, 'direct sensation is a portal to the present, whereas thought generally transports you to an imaginary past or future.'[5]

I came to realise that all of my most therapeutic moments so far, from the sober trip in California, to the harrowing truffle journey in Amsterdam, to my MDMA work, had had very little to do with words. I thought back to what Amanda Feilding had said about trauma being stuck so deep down that words can't get to it. I didn't experience childhood distress with a grown-up vocabulary or a grown-up mind, and possibly some of my trauma was pre-verbal, so how could words be the right media for soothing that distress? My therapy needed to be embodied before it was theoretical; experiential before it was explanatory.

Writers know the rule: show don't tell. If you want to make a deep and lasting emotional connection, show the audience how a character feels, don't tell them. Don't have a character tell us they're lonely. Show them sitting alone on a park bench so that the audience can feel the loneliness themselves. We are innately receptive to active, experiential learning. We don't want to be spoon-fed information, we want to be fed just enough that we can join the dots in our idiosyncratic way. It's in our nature. I'm thinking of *Jurassic Park,* and Dr Grant's observation that T-Rex doesn't want to be passively fed goat meat. T-Rex wants to hunt.[6] So much talk therapy was feeding me things that I already rationally knew, without engaging me as an embodied, feeling animal.

Trauma literature tends to favour feeling over thinking. It tends to trust the body that's grounded in reality and mistrust the mind that's lost in fiction. Since trauma theory went mainstream, it's become popular to characterise 'body knowledge' and intuition as somehow superior, even 'purer'. But we should be cautious of this dualistic hierarchy. While words can represent constriction, constraint, and inhibition, they can also be conduits to deeper connection. I would ultimately come to realise that real healing involves an integration of thinking and feeling, and a recognition that the dichotomy between the two is false.

Linguistics professors George Lakoff and Mark Johnson, in a wonderful book called *Metaphors We Live By*, suggest that language is not lofty and cerebral, but comes from the physical reality of having bodies. When we're happy, why do we say we're 'on the up', 'uplifted', and 'high on life'? Because, the authors suggest, when we're fit and well, our bodies are generally upright in space. When we dominate, why do we say we have 'control *over* someone', or we're 'on *top* of a situation'? Because in nature, larger physical bodies are often dominant. Why do we describe minds as brittle objects? 'Her ego is fragile', 'the experience shattered him', 'she snapped', etc. Because of our interactions with the properties of physical things: 'When a brittle object shatters, its pieces go flying', Lakoff reminds us, 'with possibly disastrous consequences'. Even our tendency to categorise, which I'm generally dismissive of in this book as though it were steely, clinical and unintuitive, could be thought of as expressive of our embodiment. Lakoff again: 'We impose artificial boundaries that make physical phenomena discrete just as we are: entities bounded by a surface'.[7] Maybe we see containment structures in the world because we *are* containment structures. The point is, metaphors – words that frame one concept in terms of another – are so woven into the literal fabric of who we are, we barely even notice them. But we can lean on this innate embodied imagination to heal.

During one spectacular MDMA trip in 2020, I felt a synaesthetic vision of my body rising in an incredible rush through the Earth's atmosphere at G-force speed. I was rising higher and higher, feeling more and more euphoric, when suddenly I hit a dense wall of tension, an asteroid belt of intrusive thoughts, all the content of my OCD over the years slamming into my body. I reeled through the bombardment but continued to push forward until I broke out into a wide open space of pain, where there were no more thoughts, just the endless quiet and stillness of appropriate sadness. 'Ecstatic pain' sounds like a paradox, but that's what it was: a sense of things being, though immensely difficult, in their rightful place; of coming back home into sensation that didn't have to hide itself. 'OCD is like an asteroid belt', I wrote in my notes, 'you have to get through to access pain.'

Rick Doblin, the founder of MAPS, has many times recalled how in clinical trials, participants will say something to this effect: 'I don't know why they call it ecstasy.'[8] It's important to know, if you're contemplating using this chemical, that it might not all be candy floss and fireworks. MDMA can leave you bleating and gurning like a new born wildebeest, and talking about as much sense. It's often in the most undignified moments that MDMA shows us that there is something profound about the direct experience of vulnerability, unmediated by our resistance to it. The drug brings alive the wisdom at the heart of so many psychotherapeutic traditions, and in the heart of us: that resistance to pain perpetuates it, and that surrendering to it transforms it.

The embodied metaphor of the asteroid belt gave me the physical feeling of blasting through the limiting belief that I could not effect change in the world. Through years of physical fights that I couldn't win, I'd developed a learned helplessness and mistrust of my body's power. MDMA helped me to experience what psychotherapists had been telling me for years: that I am stronger than the stories I tell about myself.

People with common mental health problems have often told me they feel trapped inside their bodies or their heads. It's a terribly lonely thing to feel – like the outside world can't be trusted to hold your emotions, which you have to keep safe inside the tiny container that is you. MDMA offers us a way to unfurl from these contracted, self-protective states and find bigger containers for our pain.

I wrote these notes during another high dose later in 2020:

Thank you, OCD. I see what you are.
I've hit a wall of confusion.
But confusion is allowed.
OCD is an illusion. What's underneath it is pain.
My OCD is a wall. I want to get through this wall.
OCD is just words. Words aren't the same as reality.
Words. Words. Words. Words. Words.
Words and doubt.
I can be with words and doubt.

My system came to a specific conclusion as I integrated these experiences: if my OCD is a protective barrier, and I'd gone to such great lengths to construct this protection, it must surely mean, as I wrote in June 2020, that 'a part of me always knew I was worth protecting'?

OCD-as-protector is a very different model to OCD-as-illness, and it was helping me in my quest to understand what had previously been a mystery to me: why I behave destructively. With this new framing, puzzling habits that I'd been told were pathological urges to hurt myself and for which I'd always hated myself (purging, cutting), started to become symptomatic not of self-destruction but of self-preservation.

Collectively, my solo MDMA experiences gave rise to a series of counterintuitive insights:

symptoms	→	strategies
tormentors	→	comforters
problems	→	attempts to solve problems
annihilation	→	survival
hate	→	love

~

Years ago, I had described the start of my anxiety in my teens as an explosion, since that was how it felt, like a sudden rush of awful feelings. But looking back, I see it as more of an implosion, a dissociation from feelings. A seizing up of a lock. A battening down of the hatches to the exclusion of emotional range. For years, my unyielding anxiety was a high, flat line:

anxious anxious anxious anxious anxious anxious anxious anxious anxious anxious

The etymological root of 'emotion' is 'moving out' or 'moving through'. We say we're 'moved by' things. It seems intuitively true that in a healthy system, emotion is free to express (press out) without constriction. Ancient Chinese medicine, with its concept of the energetic movement of *qi* throughout the body, was tapping into that intuition several

thousand years ago, often literally via acupuncture. The opposite also seems true, that mental health problems arise when
the movement of emotions is constricted.

As I had already come to understand, trauma is almost
by definition a constriction – a burial of feelings, a severance
of feelings, an escape from feelings. However you conceptualise it, the trauma response is an attempt to stop something
from happening. If we cannot, by fighting or fleeing, stop
what's going on 'out there', we can stop it in our hearts,
bury it in our guts, hide it in our minds. You may not be
able to change a situation, but you can change the emotional
projection of it. A child who is powerless to stop someone
hitting them can try to stem the emotional pain instead. A
child who is powerless to stop neglect will find some creative
way to put their shoulder to the wheel and at some level,
deep down, make their distress stop instead. Trauma is
perhaps an attempt to internally enact the power that the
external world has denied us. But this constant depression,
(pressing down), is exhausting work. As psychologist Alice
Miller wrote, 'It is precisely because a child's feelings are so
strong that they cannot be repressed without serious consequences. The stronger a prisoner is, the thicker the prison
walls have to be.'[9]

You would typically see my go-to behaviours – skin cutting,
purging, excessive drinking – represented as discrete medical
problems on separate pages of an online psychiatric resource
or in separate leaflets in the doctor's surgery. Self-harm,
bulimia, alcohol abuse. If there was cross over in the symp-
tomatology, this would be characterised as 'comorbidity', i.e.
two discrete conditions happening at the same time. This is

the systemic fragmentation of my story that I didn't realise had happened until I reviewed my mental health records and saw the historic stockpile of diagnostic labels. I believe they had prevented anyone – including Dr Harris, including me – from seeing what I would eventually come to believe: that much of what psychiatry calls 'symptoms' are functional attempts to break up the maddening stasis of trauma.

anxious anxious anxious anxious boozing anxious anxious anxious anxious anxious

anxious anxious anxious anxious anxious bingeing anxious anxious anxious anxious

anxious anxious anxious anxious anxious anxious cutting anxious anxious anxious

It's understandable that mental health care would focus on the dysfunctionality rather than the functionality of coping mechanisms, since these mechanisms can be harmful. It must be immensely challenging for a GP to assess the harm risk of a teenager with cuts on her body. It was safer for Dr Harris, during our consultation, to assume that I was still cutting than underestimate the threat I posed to myself. It is true that this kind of caution probably saves lives. It is also true that the doctor–patient dynamic demonstrated in that consultation (one of hundreds of similar encounters I had with GPs, psychiatrists and therapists), can itself give rise to insidious forms of harm.

The word 'patient' is etymologically tied up with the concept of passive suffering, of being the one who waits, of being the one who is acted upon by an external agent, being evaluated and receiving directives. The context of my psychiatric check-ups was always appraisal: *how well have you behaved for me this month? Have you abstained from doing the bad thing that we agreed you wouldn't do?* Rather than: *what riddle are you trying to solve when you cut yourself and can I support you in finding solutions?* By setting up an implicit contract under which a patient wins conditional esteem through abstention, an opportunity for compassion and insight is missed.

Rather than seeking to stamp out a person's drug or alcohol consumption and further maligning a dependency that is already deeply stigmatised, trauma expert Dr Gabor Maté asks them, as a first port of call: what did it do for you? 'Universally the answers are: it helped me escape emotional pain, gave me peace of mind, a sense of connection and a sense of control. Such responses illuminate that addiction is neither a choice nor primarily a disease. It is a forlorn attempt to solve the problem of human pain.'[10]

The *Power Threat Meaning Framework* (PTMF) is a proposed alternative to the medical model of mental health, developed in the UK in partnership with service users by a team of psychologists including Lucy Johnstone and Mary Boyle. Central to its approach is not only the consideration of what happened to a person and how this affects the meaning they make of the world, but asking what strategies they've used to survive. In the PTMF, compulsive behaviours are intelligible threat responses, not to be understood in terms of symptoms, 'but in terms of the functions they serve. These strategies arise out of core human needs to be protected, valued, find a place in the social group, and so on, and represent people's attempts, conscious and otherwise, to survive the negative impacts of power by using the resources available to them.'[11]

Cause and effect and meaning-making are also the driving force of satisfactory story, leaving room for the audience to piece together what happened and why. If motivations and consequences are too obvious and predictable, we disengage from the story. I wonder if that's part of the reason why the mental illness paradigm was so appealing to me initially and so unsatisfactory long term, because rather than empowering me to make meaning, it tried to hand it to me on a plate with a reductive explanation: 'illness is causing your suffering'.

In the *Divine Comedy*, Alighieri's fourteenth-century epic poem about a soul's journey through the afterlife, the protagonist, Dante, descends deep into the earth through nine concentric circles of hell. When Dante enters the final circle, what do you think eternal damnation looked like? Was Satan engulfed by blazing infernos? Roasting on a spit? Tormented by demons? No. Dante found Satan alone, stuck forever at the centre of a frozen lake. It's a psychologically profound image. If life is movement, hell is where nothing moves and the same beat repeats endlessly. The combustion and flickering of fire is at least energetic and therefore somehow alive. Demons are still company. In William Blake's depiction of the scene, Satan is buff with muscles he can't use and wears a crown to reign over the kingdom that immobilises him.

I hated myself every time I cut, binged or drank heavily, and doctors often added to that stigmatisation, but Alighieri's eight-hundred-year-old metaphor offers me another way to show compassion to the parts of myself that behaved compulsively and destructively. At some point, the system freezes defensively against an emotional tide and this invariability itself becomes deadening, as it always does. (If music is too ordered or predictable it doesn't sound musical. Same goes for speech: voices that lack prosody sound artificial. If you've ever seen palm plantations, where the trees have been planted uniformly in a perfect grid, it doesn't read to the brain like a forest – it seems that the chaos of a natural forest is what defines it, not just the trees.) If we see trauma as immobilisation, we might think differently about the behaviours we engage in to try to cope:

frozen frozen frozen frozen frozen frozen _{thawed} frozen frozen frozen frozen frozen frozen

The Little Match Girl by Hans Christian Andersen is a fairy tale about an impoverished child who makes a living selling matchboxes on the street. In classic Andersen style, it is grim and foreboding in tone. The little girl is cold and alone and cannot resist striking a match for warmth and light. In the flame, she sees comforting visions of the life she longs for. To keep the hope alive, she keeps striking matches, though since each match that she strikes is one she cannot sell, every little flame of comfort moves her further into destitution until she perishes. (Tomi Ungerer's adaptation[12] of the story has a much happier ending: all of her hopeful visions come true. Dad read it to me hundreds of times as a kid; I love that book.)

Writing in the mid-nineteenth century, decades before the birth of psychology as a field of study, Andersen recognised that self-destructive behaviour might counter-intuitively have comfort at its core. It's a paradox that's borne out in his creative style, which on the surface seems bleak but at its heart is deeply compassionate. We all have our little matches that we light to keep us warm, even though they lead nowhere good. Our forlorn attempts to stop pain, as Maté said: repetitive strategies that, though in the long term may alienate us, in the short term satisfy some deep universal longing for connection.

~

As I continued to work with MDMA, I started to discover a new definition for healing, one I'd grasped intellectually but never experientially, one of many I would play with over the following few years: healing as a non-resistance to pain. My trips were trying to show me that love can contain pain safely; that love won't break when you let pain into it. As if by magic, I began to feel emboldened enough to approach the painful conversation I'd been avoiding.

It came out simply one day when I was sat at dinner with my parents. The encounter had seemed enormous from far away, but like an optical illusion it was far more surmountable close up. I told them it had been difficult to watch Mom laid so low by depression and to see Dad stripped of his livelihood, and that I thought my OCD had started as a mechanism for coping with the stress of those times. They took it in, calmly and reflectively.

A few months after that, I told Dad about this book. How I thought mental health problems were largely responsive to adversities of various kinds. How I felt a sense of injustice about the way the government took his job; the way Mom was treated in hospital; the way my brother was medicated as a child. My dad has a charming, old-world habit of not feeling the need to fill silences, which means conversations with him breathe. You get the chance, in the silences, to take in your surroundings. We were walking next to a lake that afternoon. The gnats were catching the low sunlight just above the water. Dad was receptive and engaging, his insights helpful – the support that has always been a bedrock for me. We walked back to the car across the lakeshore, along the cracked banks of earth that held up the weeping willows.

It took many years for me to find a language with which to talk to my 18-year-old self, who was drinking, throwing up and cutting herself, and not understanding why. While my 'symptoms' may have looked self-annihilating from the outside and invited the disapproval of medical professionals for that reason, maybe my behaviours also showed that on some level I passionately wanted to override the stultifying trauma response and to flourish; to transcend that thick unyielding anxiety and feel things.

It's become taboo to talk about the function that acts like self-harm or purging might serve, as if to do so is to promote them. It's delicate, but I think we can explore ways, without glamorising or celebrating them, to honour the symbolic flight that they represent – the escape when no other escape is available. We can focus more on establishing feelings of safety in a person's system, less on demonising how they cope with feeling unsafe. I can see a paradoxical vitality in my reckless and regrettable behaviours, which, looking back with compassion, I view as stymied expressions of a life force that needed to move but couldn't because the mechanism was jammed. Doctors had focussed on stopping the behaviours but had rarely seen the mechanism, and when they did, they didn't have the tools to unjam it. Those, I had to go looking for.

Yes, there was a part of me, to borrow Alice Miller's metaphor, who had built thick prison walls, but perhaps there was also a part of me who was trying to break free. I wasn't sure, in 2020, which part would win out.

The invisible hand

'Because I'm undernourished, the world is a field of *getting* for me.'[1]

Rob Burbea, Buddhist scholar

When I was 22, I moved to London. I'd landed an editorial internship on the music desk of an events guide in Shoreditch that was founded, like so many media start-ups, by a pair of dazzlingly confident Eton old boys. For forty hours' work a week, they paid me £25 (the price of a weekly travel card at the time), which meant food money had to come from the dole. I skived an afternoon every two weeks to sign on at the Hoxton Job Centre, which technically was benefit fraud since my 'income' disqualified me from claiming. I slept on friends' sofas, so rent wasn't an issue. (I was tasked one day with writing a promotion for a hip-hop night called A Night Called Quest in North London. Having spectacularly misunderstood the brief, I published a bells-and-whistles announcement that hip-hop legends A Tribe Called

Quest were performing, causing the small, obscure venue to immediately oversell tickets by 1,000 per cent. I apologised profusely, but was quietly amused by the founders' anger. It was an early life lesson for me in getting what you pay for.)

I had a crush on someone in the office, a handsome coder, and also an old Etonian. After a party one night we went back to his apartment, a fancy converted factory down by the canal in Hackney, and drank whisky. He was only a year older than me, but it seemed like ten. The stories he told about the princes he'd rubbed shoulders with . . . we'd grown up in different solar systems. As we kissed on the sofa, a part of my psyche kicked out of orbit and drifted away.

'Dissociation', a severance from feelings, is one of those words that's become woolly through overuse in our psychologised pop culture, used in reference to anything from mild emotional disconnection, to hallucinating that your body is physically leaving the scene, to fugue states and atomised multiple identities. I didn't know anything about trauma back then. I hadn't yet framed my recurrent numbness as a defensive strategy of post-traumatic stress, or realised that it was also reliably triggered by any kind of sensory novelty: sudden changes in temperature, loud noises, the presence of a new person in a room. I missed the opportunity to discover all of this because I'd spent years interpreting every internal experience through a reducing valve of an idea: mental illness, a simple story that obfuscated a deeper, more complex understanding. Part of my healing would be asking myself a question: what forces, apart from my own desperate need for consolation, had led me to buy so wholeheartedly into that simple story?

~

I quickly figured out that I couldn't afford to stay in London on an editorial assistant's salary, but that I could freelance in advertising and have spare days to develop my own projects. I wanted to be a writer more than anything. When I was 23, I pitched a satirical fashion blog to the editor of *Private Eye* and got my first rejection letter: 'Good but not for us – Ed'. I still cherish that. I'd start writing *Pure* a couple of years later.

From 2010–20, I worked as a writer, then creative director, for various commercial agencies and production companies. I quickly discovered that many advertising stereotypes seemed to be true: the long boozy executive lunches in private members' clubs; the senior creative teams overwhelmingly comprised of white, public-school-educated men (according to one study[2], in 2008 only 3.6 per cent of creative directors around the world were women). From the outset, I was struck by the way that the British public was discussed in advertising agencies, as if we couldn't handle complex ideas; as if we'd lap up whatever we were served; as if our thoughts and feelings could be profiled and generalised. I didn't know that I would soon embark on a second career in mental health advocacy, or that what I was learning about the paternalistic dynamics of advertising would one day help me understand how mental health messages are shaped and sold.

The commercial industry follows a long-standing formula that has worked well since the golden age of Madison Avenue advertising in the 1960s: this product or service will make you sexier, happier, richer, better, safer. I once sat in on a meeting in a nice converted factory, in which a couple of creative directors – wearing the utilitarian clothes that manual workers wore under the same rafters a hundred years ago – tried to figure what messaging would most worry a young mother into buying baby formula. It was brazen, but there was a paradoxical honesty in the brazenness. Ad people weren't under the illusion that they were solving world hunger or promoting world peace. They were just being very good capitalists. Then the industry started to shift, as brands started to leverage social justice issues in their campaigns.

It'd started back in 2004 when skincare brand *Dove* launched their Real Beauty campaign, which set out to challenge conventional beauty standards and featured women of various body types and skin tones instead of models. By the 2010s, this style of marketing was catching on. In 2014, there was a big buzz in the industry about the Like a Girl campaign from sanitary pad brand, *Always*, which invoked the empowerment of teenage girls, featured non-actors and non-models, and barely mentioned the product itself – all recurring tropes of this new wave of 'femvertising'. In 2016, Lynx, which had always successfully traded on the message that hot women would flock towards any man who wore the deodorant, tried to reposition their image with the launch of their Find Your Magic campaign, which featured men in heels who vogued, men who said they didn't care about six packs, rebel men who ran away from riot police.

Some efforts were more toe-curling than others. There was the 2017 Pepsi commercial in which supermodel Kendall

Jenner gave a can of Pepsi to a handsome riot policeman, glaringly co-opting imagery from Black Lives Matter protests and the anti-Vietnam War campaign. On International Women's Day in 2018, a Californian branch of McDonald's turned its famous 'M' sign upside down to read as a 'W', 'in celebration of women everywhere'. Brings a tear to the eye. By the mid-to-late-2010s, so-called 'rainbow washing' was commonplace, with brands claiming to align themselves with LGBTQ+ causes by incorporating rainbow flags into their visual marketing.

Over time, my work became less about how to make a product seem irresistible but how to make the brand seem like it was caring, supportive, and liberal. Suddenly there was lots of talk about 'purpose'. Brands would spend millions engaging agencies and writers like me to define their purpose and 'authentically' signal their identity politics to audiences. You'd see the same platitudes cropping up in agency manifestos: 'we care about human connection', 'our purpose is sharing the stories that matter'. The money-counting, Scotch-drinking alpha businessmen of Madison Avenue were out. The self-proclaimed 'dreamers', 'free thinkers', and 'people who dare to do different' of new advertising were in. Cigars were out, vapes were in. Capitalism had apparently become conscious. The net result was more diverse, less misogynistic commercials. Representation matters, especially if you're from an under-represented minority.

But the problem was, representation was not reality. The change was an illusion. The advertising industry had found sanctimonious ways of repositioning its purpose, but the real purpose would always be the same: profit. I remember walking into the lobby of a huge advertising agency on International Women's Day in 2016, where an expensive floor-to-ceiling visual display showing images of famous inspiring women had been put up especially. The copy invoked the language of 'tribes': we were all one tribe; we could raise women up together. Meanwhile, at that moment, beyond the facade of this display, creative directors, the vast majority of whom were still men, were meeting with clients whose modus operandi was persuading women to buy their way out of problems like body hair, visible pores, stretch-marks, grey hair, dry hair, frizzy hair, short eyelashes and ageing. Those clients were looking for ways to liberalise their messages, but the products they were selling didn't change. Meanwhile, in a corporate culture where the client is always right (i.e. the client goes unchallenged while being as rude and demanding as they like), it was par for the course in advertising agencies to see women crying in the toilets at lunch time. All of this quite literally behind a banner of female empowerment.

Brands were becoming increasingly skilled at making you forget the gap between the scripted purpose and the actual purpose. The scripted purpose gave the illusion of progres-siveness, while still enabling the status quo to be upheld. Even while you could see the inner workings, it was easy to be beguiled by brilliant filmmaking into believing that the work was motivated by a desire to do good. It was easy to buy into the idea that the commercials of the slickest sports and tech brands were created to promote inclusivity and diversity, not to sell trainers and phones made by terribly-paid Asian factory workers.

When Shakespeare wrote *Macbeth* in around 1606, he used a metaphor to invoke the idea of concealed motives beneath surface appearances. Macbeth, who must keep his own intentions under wraps, compares nightfall to a 'bloody and invisible hand'[3]. The contradictory quality of the oxymoron adds to the scene's unsettling tone: things are not what they seem. In 1776, economist Adam Smith co-opted the metaphor, writing of 'the invisible hand'[4] of hidden, self-interested forces which drive the market and impact consumers. It can be repurposed today to describe the subtle manipulations of marketing, and the discrepancy between what the industry's doing and what it seems to be doing.

Brands may tell us that they're espousing social justice for our own good, but the invisible hand will always be working underneath to its own ends, nudging us to consume. In its paternalism and tokenism, advertising routinely reduces complex issues to surface-level representations, to advance a story that serves an industrial purpose. Perhaps you're starting to get a sense of why I think all of this is relevant to the mental health industry.

~

Dr Derek Summerfield is one of the most charismatic and articulate critical psychiatrists I've encountered. He's worked extensively in poverty-stricken and war-torn populations around the world, and takes a dim view of the export of Western ideas about psychology and psychiatry into non-Western cultures, which he sees as a kind of medical imperialism that subjugates local knowledge and practices. When I met Dr Summerfield at a conference about global mental health[5], he told me that the '1:4' statistic (the often-quoted stat that one in four people in the world have a mental illness), was 'bullshit', because there's no global definition or objective measurement of mental illness.

By 2018, I had collaborated with many charities and had co-founded a mental health non-profit.

I'd frequently used the '1:4' statistic to justify the fight against stigma. I wanted mental illnesses to be globally recognised as illnesses like any other. My meeting with Dr Summerfield had catalysed my ongoing process of personal reckoning with the messages I was spreading. Was '1:4' true? And if not, how and why had I come to believe that it was?

The statistic seemed to be a composite, an estimate drawn from many sources: some considered lifetime prevalence of mental health problems; some considered prevalence in a year; all took for granted that a mental problem was something that could be externally defined and measured; none specified which parts of the world had and hadn't been studied.

I came across a 2014 BBC radio debate between Martin Seager, a consultant clinical psychologist, and Sue Baker, the former director of Time to Change, the most influential mental health campaign of the last two decades.

Martin argued that the use of '1:4' as a slogan was a mistake because it implied that mental health problems were something that you either have or you don't, obscuring the fact that we're all on a spectrum.

Sue Baker disagreed. She argued that '1:4' has served to normalise mental illness and has played an important part in changing public attitudes, 'We did think about the "everyone-has-mental-health-and-we're-all-on-a-spectrum" messages, but they weren't working with the general public when we tested them. What worked better was the fact that they didn't know much about mental health . . . and they didn't realise that people face stigma and discrimination.'[6]

My ears pricked up. Slogans, campaigns, messaging, user testing. This was a language I understood because I used it every day to shape stories for brands. I'd been able to see clearly how advertisers were using social justice causes to nudge audiences. It dawned on me, as I listened to this piece, that the osmosis was going in the other direction: social justice causes were also using the machinery of advertising.

'The Time to Change campaign is doing more good than harm, of course,' Martin said. 'But it could do more good if it stressed the point that mental health is something we *all* have.'

'I think it's important to state that we're starting with baby steps', Sue said, 'where the general population, over so many generations, has been so discriminatory towards those of us who have mental health problems. We are just beginning. At the bottom of a very big mountain to climb. Ideally, we'd want everybody to realise that we're all on this spectrum and that mental health is an issue for every human being, but getting to that point is going to take time. It may be that the campaign does move on creatively, when the public are ready to move on.'

'No, I disagree with that one,' Martin said. 'I think it's slightly patronising to the public to think that they don't "get" mental health. I think if it was packaged in a way that made sense in their real lives, they would get it.'

Then Martin announced that he'd written some alternative

campaign messaging that he thought might be more relatable to audiences and proceeded to read it aloud:

You don't have mental health issues if you've never experienced any of the following:

If you weren't rejected, neglected, hurt or badly misunderstood by the adults responsible for you when you were growing up. If you never experienced favouritism at home, school or work. If you never experienced bullying at home, school or work. If you never felt like an outsider. If you never looked in the mirror and felt unattractive. If you never got betrayed or hurt in a love relationship. If you never comforted yourself with substances, food, drink, gambling or similar. If you never experienced traumatic loss of something much loved – a person, a dream or a job. If you never pretended or fantasised that you were more special or important than you felt yourself to be. If you never felt terror of failure, death, illness or rejection. If you never doubted the point of your existence or wished you weren't here. If you never felt devalued or put down because of your looks, your accent, your class, your nationality, your gender or religion. . . These are all mental aspects of the human condition, not mental conditions.'[7]

Tears ran down my cheeks. I hadn't realised the extent to which the messaging of my advocacy had been divisive; how it had separated us (the one in four), from everyone else (the three in four). Us with a disease, them without one.

(As we've seen, I also agree with the counterargument that

framing mental health as a spectrum issue can trivialise the suffering of the most seriously distressed. But I don't think that drawing arbitrary lines and labelling some people as having mental illnesses necessarily gets them the help they need, or that they're inevitably harmed if others at the milder end of the spectrum identify with their problems.)

My puzzle about the forces that'd led me to view mental health in medicalised terms had spilled out of academia and onto my turf: marketing. I had presumed that '1:4' was a factual communication of the reality of our mental health landscape, and that spreading awareness of this was comparable to sharing other useful public health messages, like excessive alcohol increasing the risk of liver disease. But though it had been presented as fact, '1:4' seemed to be more like a strapline that served to steer audiences towards a subjective medicalised world view.

Back in the room, Sue Baker replied, 'I do agree with what Martin is saying about looking at mental health as a life issue . . . But I do have to say, it's a quantum leap to expect the public to see that everybody has mental health, in the same way that they have physical health . . . We are years away from the public thinking like that.'[8]

Who gets to decide when the public is ready to hear how mysterious and little understood mental health is? Do charities get to decide? Policy makers? Doctors? To me there was something troubling about questioning our readiness at all. I'd seen paternalism at work in advertising. There, the intention had been profit, while here, the intention was fighting stigma, but the methodology was similar. Both ran on the assumption that the public were not ready for complex ideas, that we needed to be spoon-fed carefully managed stories, and that certain groups of people have the authority to do the management on our behalf.

In 2023, I'd call Sue Baker to find out if her views had changed.

'You've previously said that you didn't think the public was ready to hear more nuanced perspectives on mental health. Do you think they're ready now?'

'Back in the day, our frame of reference for mental health was the "mad asylum on the hill",' Sue said. 'The community does have to be ready and educated. You can't fight for people's rights unless you transform society's attitudes. We took a solid social marketing behaviour-change approach. You assess what you need to say to people next, to take them on a journey of not just thinking differently but changing their behaviour. We needed to work on stigma before another campaign could come along and say "It's 4:4 – we all have mental health".'

'Could medicalised messages, ironically, create more stigma?' I asked.

'We did start to see emerging evidence that messaging like "mental illness is like any other" can actually be counterproductive.[9] People with lived experience know that it's not like any other illness, is it? So we ended up not using that any more, we were careful to avoid it.'

'Do you think that people have an intuitive understanding of mental health?'

'People have more information now, yes. Still probably quite a limited frame of reference: you get sick, you go to the doctor, you get medication or therapy. Do people really understand that how you live your life impacts your mental health? They might not use mental health language, but I think they're aware of how it's making them feel. I definitely see more people seeking help, even if it's not the right kind of help.'

'It's obvious that the work you've done has been beneficial in a way. When my mom was given a diagnosis of bipolar disorder, campaigns like yours were comforting,' I said. 'But medicalised messages can also stop people getting the right kind of help.'

'I do agree we need to take a much more systemic approach to preventing distress in the first place by trying to deal with the underlying causes. If a woman has poor housing and mould on the walls and children to feed, and there isn't a way of changing her circumstances, then what do we do? Leave that person to struggle? I know this approach is limited but the bigger policy problems are still not solved.'

'It's so difficult to know what to do, isn't it?' I said. 'My concern is that medicalised narratives, which I spread myself in my advocacy, can be attractive to policymakers because they shift the burden of responsibility on to psychiatrists and individuals.'

'If you put a mental health lens on every piece of government policy, we'd all be in a much better place, right? I could have easily been side-tracked with these major issues, but I had a mandate to transform attitudes. I needed to keep us on the rail tracks and focus. I think if we had taken on that task, we would have confused an already confused public at the outset.'[10]

I agree with Sue that the issues are major and complex,

and that stigma is a problem. It's a problem especially for those with psychosis and for Black people with mental health problems, who are almost five times more likely to be detained under the Mental Health Act than white people.[11]

But I think stigma is where our problems seep to the surface. It is not anywhere near the source of our mental health crisis. I think we tackle mental health at the level of stigma because we are desperate to help and we don't know what else to do. But I'd say the onus of responsibility should be less on the public to change their attitudes, and more on those who govern to change their policies. And yes, it's progress that the 'asylum on the hill' trope has been rescinded, but sanitised versions of those institutions still exist. We don't call it madness, we call it mental illness. But we still lock people up and tie them down, with chemical restraints if not physical ones.

This conversation points to the siloed nature of our response to the mental health crisis – it is hard to take a step back and look at the whole picture. It also points to the problems that arise when we seek to demystify issues that can't be easily reduced.

In the mental health conversation, the public's confusion is frequently invoked as a justification for simplified stories; stories that, in the long run, contribute further to people's confusion. Of course we need easy-to-understand messages, but I don't think people are as resistant to complexity as those working in media often believe. Nor do I think that gatekeeping knowledge is helpful. If the public doesn't know that the message they're receiving is reductive, yet those dispensing the message do, that gap strikes me as being at odds with what's central to collective healing: trust, openness to ambiguity, and authentic connection.

We are living through an authenticity crisis, in part because we've let the tools of marketing shape the issues we care about most. In the 2010s, it wasn't just charities that were using advertising tactics; individuals were also starting to behave like brands through the rise of influencer marketing. Charismatic people who were devoted to certain social justice causes and who had large social media followings would be paid to promote brands while they were raising awareness. It started to become normal to see, for example, body positivity influencers promoting underwear brands, or mental health influencers promoting therapy apps. Sometimes it was hard to know if you were engaging with a human being or a product, or some new emergent blend of both. *Is this post really about 'awareness' or is it primarily serving some other purpose? A career? A content quota? A need for validation and love?* A strategist I know at a massive creative agency, who finds social media influencers to amplify mental health awareness, told me, sardonically, that their 'entire job is giving people opportunities for vanity'.

In the wake of *Pure,* I frequently received offers for collaborations from companies in fast fashion, CBD, and digital therapeutics (chatbots, wearables, app-based therapy, etc.). Here's one of the messages:

> On your profile, you mention you are researching psychedelics, consciousness and trauma. [My company] specialises in DISSOLVING TRAUMA. We are looking to collab with people who would be interested in healing sessions and then in return share the experience with their followers.

It's a familiar formula: we'll reward you if you spread a simple story – 'trauma can be dissolved' – that will lead people to a purchase decision. These kinds of transactions are commonplace; indicative of the mutual back scratching that is happening across psychiatry and therapy; and demonstrative of the hidden forces that influence how we spend our healing dollars. (I declined the offer, by the way; they weren't to know that I don't get out of bed for anything less than a lifetime's supply of super-absorbent menstrual pants.)

As brands leverage reductive and tokenistic stories of identity, so too does the mental health industry. In a world of hourly therapy rates, pay-per-view film launches, conferences with three-figure price tags, sponsored posts, and trademarked therapeutic modalities, it's helpful if we are separated into atomised and clearly signposted consumer groups: people with diagnoses; people with trauma; survivors. We often find ourselves following these signposts because we're looking for a place to belong.

In recent years we've seen the memetic rise of 'my lived experience'. The phrase is helpful in shining a light on the intrinsic validity of each person's interpretation of themselves, but it is often used to shut down conversation rather than open it up. Each person's lived experience is inseparable from the lived experiences of everyone around them, but this is not a commercially helpful story.

Psychiatry generally ignores that disrupted human connection is almost always at the heart of mental health problems. That so-called symptoms are almost always some kind of misfiring attempt to get that connection back; that human connection is our way out of suffering, and that if any theory, therapy or chemical intervention works, they work not in and of themselves, but because they are conduits to human connection.

Instead, it triages us along medical lines, because, it says, I have a diagnosis of OCD and you have a sex addiction, because I compulsively ruminate and you compulsively fawn, because I have a history of self-harm and you have a history of calorie-restriction. Over-working, overspending, over-exercising? Aggression or passive aggression? Maybe you can't stop taking selfies, or you can't stop cheating. Maybe the slightest insult triggers your rage, or you have no sexual confidence. Maybe your strategies are more somatic than psychological and take the form of any number of stress-immune responses and idiopathic health conditions, for which you'll get annexed to a whole different branch of medicine. Us over here getting prescribed antidepressants; you over there getting prescribed steroids. Industrial medicine is not incentivised to take a step back and consider what we might all have in common.

Alexander Beiner, author of the book *The Bigger Picture*, about psychedelics' potential to improve the world, put it well: 'Hype can make it appear as though we understand what's causing this [mental health] crisis. We don't. From the perspective of biomedical psychiatry, our depressions, anxieties and addictions can be fixed with the right drugs. From another perspective, this crisis is a desperate howl from the heart of consumer culture.'[12]

Many well-meaning advocacy and treatment efforts from many talented, compassionate people over many decades, have statistically failed to improve mental health generally. Perhaps that's because we're trying to heal with the same tools that make us howl, and because healing itself has become an individualistic consumerist culture. Even when they are backed by rigorous science, the mainstream explanatory models for why we suffer and what works (the biomedical model, the trauma model, the psychedelics-as-medicines model), spread like brand stories, shaped by the invisible hand of commercial incentives. In my view, the best thing sufferers can do in the healing marketplace is cultivate our media literacy and scepticism, and take a pluralistic, promiscuous approach when contemplating which stories and labels best capture our experience. We are harder to market to if we are irreducible.

As without, so within

'Birth begins the process of learning to be separate. The separation is hard to believe or accept. Yet, as we accept it our imagination grows – imagination which is the capacity to reconnect, to bring together, that which is separate. Metaphor finds the traces which indicate that all is one. Acts of solidarity, compassion, self-sacrifice, generosity, are attempts to re-establish – or at least a refusal to forget – a once-known unity.'[1]

John Berger, novelist

A black Audi with tinted windows waits in the carpark. It's dark out and the car is conspicuous with its lights on. I walk over and the door is opened from the inside. I don't like getting into dealers' cars. With my beating heart and tense stomach, my nervous system is reminding me of what we're told by society from the moment we're cognisant: don't speak to strangers; and definitely, especially as a woman, don't get into strangers' cars. I go against my gut, get in, hand the dealer £50 for a gram of MDMA, and leave as quickly as possible.

An hour after taking a bomb of it the next day, I throw a cushion across the room and shout in frustration. It's early 2021, and there has been no good MDMA on the streets of London for a few months since the lockdown ban on partying caused a slump in imports from Europe. This is my second dud batch – no psychoactive effects – and my second thwarted session. I sit on the bedroom floor, clenching my fists. I don't know if I can do this any more. Every avenue that I try, access is blocked. I cannot get through. Nothing has ever got through. Self-help did not get through. Psychotherapy did not get through. Antidepressants did not get through. Rationality did not get through. Kind words do not get through. *I* cannot get through. I've lost count of how many solo MDMA sessions I've done. I've had a lot of profound insights but something is not translating. The insights are slipping through my fingers and I don't know why.

I roll onto my side and start shivering. I shouldn't be here alone like this, taking risks with my health like this – fuck knows what I've just ingested. But if the sound advice and healing community that I need exists, I don't know how to find it. Fuck, I'm anxious. I look it up. The crystals were probably made up of so-called 'imposter substances' like 4-CMC or eutylone, that cause mild psychoactive effects and can cause anxiety, but aren't dangerous in these dosages. I need water and rest. But I'm ruminating too much to sleep, so I scribble furiously in my notebook.

If trauma is blocking off access to pain, then society colludes in the blocking. For years, the health system, with its unscientific pathologisation of my suffering, has blocked access to a holistic account of my life. Now, the government's categorisation of MDMA and psilocybin as drugs with 'no therapeutic value' is blocking my access to safe psychedelic healing. As within, so without. I think about what Amanda Feilding said to me a couple of years before, about society being a projection of what's inside us. Yes, and maybe it goes the other way too. Maybe what's inside us is a projection of society. Maybe internal fragmentation reflects external fragmentation, and the psychological and physiological repression of trauma is an internal projection of a society-wide repression of pain, a subconscious desire to keep half of the picture hidden. Maybe that's why our mental health system is so unbelievably fucked: not because of lies, or conspiracy, or because anyone's greedy or bad, but because pain is hard, and it's easier to cut pain off, intellectualise it and put it in boxes, than it is to feel it. The biomedical model disconnects us from our stories, trauma disconnects us from our stories. Drug laws suppress free expression, trauma suppresses free expression. Access is denied, access is denied. As without, so within.

I'm glad I can see that tree out of my window; the twists and crossings of the branches are more chaotic than what's in my head. I can't see the trunk for the plumes of dark green ivy that is slowly taking over. One arm of it reaches skywards exuberantly and is almost at the uppermost branches. My Palaeolithic counterpart would've known what species of tree it was, whether its berries were edible and what the leaning of its branches said about the weather. Magpies nested last year, two for joy. I hope they'll be back.

I'm not just lonely, I'm existentially lonely. I've felt like this a lot since I got into psychedelics. Like I never knew how ardently I was longing for connection until I felt the longing and now it can't be put back.

I rest my head on a cushion and look up at the bookshelf. There's plenty of solace up there, too; no emotion I could feel that hasn't already been felt on those pages. The confused little monkey on the cover of John Berger's *Why Look at Animals?* looks down at me like a mirror. The book is a philosophical essay about our relationship with the natural world. In zoos, Berger posits that we don't just cage animals, we cage the part of us that knows we are not separate from them. We imprison that part because the knowledge of loss that it bears is too painful to unleash.[2]

If zoos are a monument to the disappearance of what Berger beautifully calls a 'once-known unity',[3] maybe trauma is a monument to humans' lost connection to each other, caging us off because contemplating that bygone unity is too painful. If imagination, the bringing together of disparate elements, is the antidote to disunity, maybe it's an antidote to trauma too. Maybe our ability to imagine how things could be different is the tinder that ignites transformation.

It was only when I got into psychedelics that I began to see the ways in which my great life, with its dining out and professional accolades and holidays in the calendar, was, at bottom, unfulfilling. How often do I help people less fortunate than me in practical ways? Almost never. How often do I hold hands with friends or lie around with them like the apes that we are? Rarely. What spaces of learning and community do I attend where I know I'll see people I love (not including work, where I'm paid to be, or the pub, where alcohol depresses my mood and affects my sleep)? None.

In the West we have lost almost all of our collective outlets for processing pain. No initiation ceremonies. No threshold rites to mark the turning of life stages. No ritualistic offerings or cleanses, no formalised solitude or dark nights of the soul. No social procedures or structures to facilitate affirmation, forgiveness, gratitude, or grief. Very little collective singing beyond church. Very little collective dancing beyond clubs. I'm so disconnected from these kinds of traditions that modern attempts to recreate them often make me cringe. It all seems so hippie or lame or cultish. Where does that judgement come from? Why are so many of us closed off to the idea of ritualistically exploring emotion? Maybe because deep down we know the immense upheaval involved in truly meeting ourselves. It makes sense, in a world that offers little social support for that upheaval, that we would be allergic to going anywhere near our feelings. It's perhaps even wise and self-protective not to want to undertake the task.

I once heard a simple explanation for our mental health crisis: everything that we used to do as cooperative groups of adults, we now do alone, or in tiny contained units. Gathering food, cooking food, eating food, bathing, playing, travelling, working. Almost all our problems have to be solved not by committee but in our minds. But maybe some problems, or even most problems, cannot be solved there. I decide that afternoon that I'm not going to do MDMA alone any more.

The question that I asked earlier: how can you know what happened to you and *not know* at the same time? I tried to answer it with a bio-psychological explanation: my brain and body was repressing access to knowledge. But there are social repressors too. Maybe we struggle to join the dots in our own hearts because society makes it difficult, not by design but because of the imperatives and incentives of the way we live. You're not chipping away at your sales targets if you're drinking psychoactive brews in the jungle. You're not on deadline if you're sitting in silence. You're not being productive if you're taking time out to reconnect with family.

If we rediscover our bodies' connectedness to everything around us, that's potentially quite radical and disruptive, since it points to the uncomfortable truth that most of what we do in consumer society runs counter to our happiness. If we 'refuse to forget', as Berger put it, our once-known unity,[4] we might refuse to participate in things as they are.

Rock

In 1945, around the
time that my French
grandparents fell preg-
nant with my mother
(shortly after Papy
André escaped from his
Nazi captors), a
17-year-old English girl
called Betty Farley got
a surprise: she was preg-
nant. She worked as a
screw machinist in a
factory in Birmingham.
She was poor and
unwed, and the father
had disappeared. Betty
went to a mother-and-
baby home run by
nuns and gave birth to
a boy: my dad. At the
time, a tacit forced
adoption policy shamed
and pressured young
mothers into giving
'illegitimate' children
up for adoption. When
Betty tried to return
home with her new
baby, her parents
turned her away, giving
her no choice but to
leave him with a local
Catholic orphanage.
The nuns later recalled
how Betty showered
him with love every
day when she came in
to breastfeed him.

Healing in three acts

'For me, mythology is a function of biology . . . a product of the soma's imagination. What do our bodies say? And what are our bodies telling us? The human imagination is grounded in the energies of the body.'[1]

Joseph Campbell, mythologist

You never forget your first counsellor. Mine was a small, bearded man with long, grey hair and a kind face, who seemed ancient but was probably no older than 40. I was 18 years old. It was that first year of university when Mom had once again gone up Bushey Fields, when I was self-harming and throwing up my meals. My GP, Dr Harris, had prescribed a course of sessions alongside the antidepressants.

I saw my new counsellor late afternoon once a week in the loft of a Victorian terrace, all sloping walls and wood chip. Really more of a crawl space than a room, but I found its smallness comforting. The only window was a skylight. The counsellor, always focussed, always listening, would sit in the silver air underneath it and slowly disappear like a druid in the mist until he put the lamps on.

At the end of our final session, I gave him a gift: a jazz CD. I've never bought a therapist a present since and I still don't know if it's appropriate. It struck me as extraordinary and cool that a stranger would listen to you talk for an hour or so about whatever you wanted, since I was fresh out of school where I'd spent a decade and a half being told to shut up. He'd never expressed any interest in jazz, but I guess I thought that's what old people listened to. He seemed touched by the gesture, if a little bemused. Maybe he'd forgotten the hushed, adolescent language of a mixtape, of massive incomprehensible feelings ferried in track numbers from one bustling heart to another. I liked track three and hoped he'd like it too. The flute was wizardy and reedy like him. That CD must now be stacked at the back of an Oxfam somewhere, or stowed in a musty cellar, or regifted to an enemy, perhaps. But the gift he gave me when he slipped a piece of paper into my hands with a 'good luck', never became obsolete.

It was an extract from a book by Carl Rogers, a very famous American psychologist I'd never heard of. I read it at the bus stop on the way back from therapy:

I remember that in my boyhood, the bin in which we stored our winter's supply of potatoes was in the basement, several feet below a small window. The conditions were unfavourable, but the potatoes would begin to sprout – pale, white sprouts, so unlike the healthy green shoots they sent up when planted in the soil in the spring. But these sad, spindly sprouts would grow 2 or 3 feet in length as they reached toward the distant light of the window. The sprouts were, in their bizarre, futile growth, a sort of desperate expression of the directional tendency I have been describing. They would never become plants, never mature, never fulfil their real potential. But under the most adverse circumstances, they were striving to become. Life would not give up, even if it could not flourish. In dealing with clients whose lives have been terribly warped, in working with men and women on the back wards of state hospitals, I often think of those potato sprouts. So unfavourable have been the conditions in which these people have developed that their lives often seem abnormal, twisted, scarcely human. Yet, the directional tendency in them can be trusted. The clue to understanding their behaviour is that they are striving, in the only ways that they perceive as available to them, to move toward growth, toward becoming. To healthy persons, the results may seem bizarre and futile, but they are life's desperate attempt to become itself.[2]

The obvious message of the extract is resilience in darkness, but I had not yet understood its deeper meaning, or what the wizard was encouraging me to think about when he gave me that bit of paper. I was so cut off from any sense of the cause and effect of my own life that I didn't see the relevance. But I think on some level I was responding, because as I read it, the piece of paper was quivering in my hands.

~

In early 2021, a few months after I'd vowed to stop doing solo MDMA sessions, I tapped into a network of trustworthy underground psychedelics guides working in the UK. My first guided MDMA session happened in early summer of that year at the house of two guides, Rachel and Jonathan.

I had no idea how this was going to pan out. In my solo MDMA sessions I'd expressed huge emotions, but I was an expert at not showing my feelings to others. When I was a kid, I'd kept my distress to myself for a few interrelated reasons. According to trauma theory, I was unconsciously repressing that distress. Certainly, I was consciously trying to keep my head down so as not to make a stressful family predicament more stressful. I was, at least until I discovered miniskirts and alcopops, as fawning, studious, and polite as possible in an attempt to keep the peace. I did not show my emotions.

The phrase 'holding space' has become somewhat clichéd. It means a physical space, somewhere safe and free from interruption, prepped with whatever lighting, interiors, and music is most conducive to your aims. But there's an emotional dimension to it too. If space is held for you, you are accepted as you are, your emotions are welcomed without judgement or over-reactivity. You are encouraged to explore your psyche, safe in the understanding that you'll be met with a response that is comforting, commensurate, and empathetic, from someone whose nervous system is soothed, grounded, and capacious. In a space like this you can, within reason, let go. You can scream, you can cackle, you can gurgle and punch pillows, you can sigh in bliss or yell in anger.

Another related complication of the fawn response is that, because you hide your distress, you never get the chance to see your distress reflected back at you in the faces of others – the validating mirror that says these feelings exist. If you refuse to show vulnerability, you never get to map the wrench in your heart onto the furrowed brow of a witness, or the knots in your stomach onto the tightened facial muscles of their pout. These self-stymying tactics, and the resulting lack of opportunity for validation, can have the net effect of making your emotional life feel unreal, and of limiting your expressive range. Various therapists remarked over the years that I had what they call a 'flat affect', i.e. a lack of reaction to emotional stimuli, and an expressionless face when I was talking about very distressing subjects. We cannot break out of this crushing solipsism without recruiting other people as witnesses.

On the morning of my first guided trip with Rachel and Jonathan, after a herbal tea and a chat, I took my first dose, a little bomb of MDMA in tissue paper, put on the eye mask and lay down.

Rachel kept these notes during the journey:

11.45
First dose.
Quiet couple of hours.

13.45
Second dose.
'I'm swimming in loneliness.'

14.20
More of the same.
'Struggling to push through the frustration while sensing it's important to feel the feelings.'
'Not felt them with such intensity before.'

15.30
'Some of the tension has passed, it feels a bit easier.'

16.00
Directed by Rose, Jonathan stroked her hair and Rachel held her hand.

16.30
Gentle rocking.

When I read Rachel's notes back, I was surprised to learn that the first couple of hours had seemed quiet from the outside. On the inside, I'd been very busy.

As I'd come up, I'd felt my ego split in two, into my child-self who felt sick with fear, and my adult-self who was coaching her through that fear. I had the sense of my entire childhood rushing past as I stayed suspended in this dyadic self; reliving my life as both the worried kid and the grown-up supporting her. The kid didn't speak, but she could hear and understand the adult's reassurances: 'Whatever's out there, I'll be with you, you'll be okay.' The osmosis went two ways. The adult could feel the kid's pain: 'This was too much for you to bear, I see that now.' The kid seemed comforted to know that she'd been seen and that she wasn't alone any more. Shored up by that lifetime's worth of pep-talking, I was now ready to dive into an ocean of previously unfelt feelings. That's where you see me verbalise at the two-hour mark: 'I'm swimming in loneliness.'

What struck me more than anything about Rachel's observations, which mapped neatly onto my phenomenology, was the narrative shape. The trip read like a story. There was a beginning preparatory phase, a middle confrontation phase, and a final integration phase. I had the strange feeling of having moved through this structure many times in my solo sessions despite never having noticed it before.

I looked back through the last two years of notebooks. They had followed the pattern without fail. The content and qualia of the experiences had varied – sometimes they were more blissful, sometimes more harrowing, but the form seemed consistent.

Act one, usually lasting up to ninety minutes, was a departure from ordinary consciousness in a rush of energy, sheathed with enough soothing to deliver me into act two, an epic two-to-three hour transformation via confrontation (a memory, a mysterious sensory landscape, a feared idea). Act three was a lower octane trip back to the surface as lessons from the beyond were integrated into the here and now. It seemed to follow what Joseph Campbell called the monomyth[3], our universal story: departure, initiation, and return. Departure, when the protagonist is presented with their challenge and prepared for their journey; initiation, when they cross into another realm and overcome transformative challenges; return, when they re-enter their world of origin having brought something back from the beyond.

The following notes are from back in July 2019 – only the second MDMA solo therapeutic trip that I did:

As I come up. Aware of bodily anxiety. Tolerate it.
It's allowed to be there. I don't have to be afraid. But I am.
This is about my body.

There is blockage. I feel the blockage. Notice the blockage. Love is complicated for me because it wasn't easy. The blockage is powerful. Thicker, deeper, heart racing. Swimming through dark pool. In my chest. My worst fear, the distillate. I've seen the core.

You can let it go.

And this is an account from a trip I did in May 2021:

Coming up, feeling great. The past is in the present. Nothing more to worry about. I feel like it's gone. It's all in the past.

Twenty solid minutes of awful desolation.

I accept all parts of myself. I don't have to control any thoughts or feelings.

It also seemed to be there in how others described their MDMA experiences to me, and in accounts I read in books and online. My guide confirmed that she'd seen this pattern in other clients too. Preparation on the way up, a series of transformative encounters at the peak, an insight on the way down.

As soon as I'd noticed it, I brushed off the observation. Hardly surprising that a writer would spot a writerly pattern, and besides, insights from psychedelic experiences, like so much in psychology, are best grasped lightly. As I mentioned before, you can run into trouble if you interpret psychedelic phenomena too literally or rush to conclusions before they've had a chance to bed in, if they ever do. It's also okay for psychedelic experiences to remain unintegrated, bizarre, ungraspable, and free from any imposed meaning.

What's more, I have OCD, which means that over-association and over-learning are some of my core psychological mechanics. My system has developed a survival tactic of repeatedly overinterpreting meaning to the exclusion of novel information, so I've learned to mistrust my own conclusions.

Psychology and cognitive science professor John Vervaeke has spoken at length about how anxious people's tendency for pattern recognition can keep them from truth rather than lead them to it: 'The very machinery that makes you adaptive is the machinery that makes you prey to self-deception'.[4] In other words, if we're constantly on the lookout for safety or threat, we tend to see salience where there is none. That's why I try to underwrite my conclusions about my mental health with frequent reminders of my own capacity for bullshit.

But no matter how much I tried to dismiss the comparison between the structure of healing processes and the three-act structure, there seemed to be something in it. It would not stop knocking on my door, emerging not just through my MDMA work, but across a range of altered states of consciousness: preparation, confrontation, integration.

~

In 2019, off the back of my psilocybin trip in Amsterdam and my first couple of solo experiments with MDMA, I'd wanted to start psychotherapy again to help me integrate those experiences. The knot in my chest seemed to be nudging me with intuitions: *keep going, keep going, keep going.* I'd sought out a therapist with an interest in complex trauma, and someone qualified to practise EMDR, a kind of embodied psychotherapy that stands for Eye Movement Desensitisation and Reprocessing.

In EMDR's classic form, a therapist asks a client to follow alternate flashing lights with their eyes. Strangely, this rapid alternating activation of the left and right hemispheres seems to cause the client to drop into a trancelike state in which they have vivid visuals or sensations, thought to be memories, which they are then able to 'reprocess', i.e. re-experience in a new, safe context. (According to the REM hypothesis of EMDR, the technique's bilateral stimulation shifts the brain into a memory processing mode similar to that of REM sleep, when your eyes rapidly move left to right.)

I'd been drawn to therapist Joyce Blake after an initial phone call. We got on well and seemed to have similar sensibilities. She'd been a journalist in a previous career and was interested in the role of creativity and play in healing. Like almost all of the therapists I'd chosen in the past, she was also, not coincidentally, old enough to be my mother.

I noticed a three-act structure in this work, too. Joyce would begin a session with preparatory resourcing: a body scan and a visualisation of a safe place, to ensure that I was grounded, secure, and prepared to 'go there'. This would be followed by the processing part of the session, in which I approached difficult memories or sensations while bilateral stimulation took place. Towards the end, enough time would be allowed for me to slowly return from whatever intense psychological phenomena I'd encountered back into the present moment, with re-orientating mindfulness exercises: 'name five things you can see', 'pay attention to your feet on the ground', etc. By way of denouement, we'd then talk about whatever had come up.

The structure had also appeared in a body psychotherapy I'd started the following year called craniosacral therapy. My therapist, Peter Buckoke, would begin by holding my feet and encouraging me to take deep breaths. He would then place his palms on my head or back, or mobilise my limbs, somehow mysteriously triggering an altered state of consciousness, and the expression through my body via shakes, stretches, punches or kicks, of deep emotion, until it reached a point of natural resolution. I'd been sceptical of this kind of healing because of all of those 'trauma release' viral videos of people shaking and wailing, which for me typified a worrying new trend of turning trauma into bitesize content opportunities. And because craniosacral is often dismissed by doctors as a pseudoscience. Yet when I'd tried it, I'd found it nothing less than profound. It's unclear to me how its subjective effects (the feeling that energy is moving in your body, the strange sense of *being* your younger self) could be captured by current scientific methods. I wrote this note about a session in October 2021:

When Peter put his hands on my head, I started to feel the awful tug of trying to let go and trying to hold on at the same time . . . He started moving my legs. At first they were sluggish and didn't do anything. Then they wanted to kick out. He contained the kicking. I was rageful as I kicked against his hands. I arched my back and tensed while I kicked. Then I broke into massive sobs and went limp.

You can sense the rhythm of a story in the build of muscle tension, followed by the emotional release and drop off. Whether through MDMA, EMDR or body work, there was always a drop off – a point of completion, a sense of having done whatever could be done for the time being and of returning to base for rest. There was a musicality to it. It was like what bassist Bootsy Collins called the basic funk formula[5]: do whatever you want in between the first beats of each bar, as long as you get back to 'the one'.

Perhaps my body's healthy instinct for self-protection had been stymied by the constant physical fighting during my childhood, but with the help of skilled therapists, who trusted that somewhere this instinct was still intact, I was able express the emotions that got locked up a long time ago with my bracing muscles. I started to see therapy less like an external intervention and more like a catalyst for internal processes that already have the potential to unfold; a relationship that facilitates your idiosyncratic way of healing.

Remember, as you surf through the dizzying array of trademarked therapies which all put some shiny, new, never-before-seen framework behind a catchy acronym and paywall, Dumbo didn't need the feather. And yet he did need a helper. It was only with the support of Timothy Mouse that he could transform his rather large problems into his salvation. The things that keep us down, as the wise mouse counselled Dumbo, are the very things which can lift us up.[6]

As my system was guided through this timeless structure

again and again, I fondly remembered the wizard and the Carl Rogers extract, which I'd cherished and kept in a shoebox under the bed. Holding it in my steady hands eighteen years later, I understood it in a visceral way, since by then I had the experience that matched the theory. I was waking up to my own directional tendency, to that bit of me that had always been pushing forwards towards becoming, like potato shoots in the dark.

~

I wondered if I was getting to the heart of the mysterious quality that's alluded to by the trauma-healing clichés of 'the body knows what to do', 'trust your inner healing intelligence', and 'unleash your inner healing wisdom'. As your skin independently knows how to repair when you graze yourself, maybe there was a comparable psychospiritual mechanism that somehow 'knows' how to join the dots, and that, given the right conditions, will always evolve in the right direction. 'Evolve' comes from the Latin *evolvere*, meaning 'unfolding', 'unrolling' or, interestingly, 'the opening of a book'. Come to think of it, 'story' is almost a synonym of directionality, and creativity is almost a synonym of integration: bringing together what is separate. I've never heard an account of healing that didn't involve both.

Yes, it seemed increasingly plausible to me that the mystery of how we understand stories is the mystery of how we heal, since their essence is the same: moving towards wholeness. Both processes seem to speak to what Rogers described as 'life's attempt to become itself'[7]. But an unconscious attempt? How could that be possible? How does the body *know what to do*? How does it, in Bessel van der Kolk's framing, keep the score? Science has only given a partial answer.

In a wonderful short book called *Myth and the Body*, psychologist Stanley Keleman and mythologist Joseph Campbell argue that story is innate in us, since our bodies physically and inescapably bear the hallmark of story, just by existing. We are born, we live, and we die:

Our bodies, our somatic and emotional processes, have a beginning, a middle ground, and an end, that give our structure and imaginative functions a coherency. Mythology is structured in the cells. Each sperm cell, each egg, contains a story that is recreated in the full growth of each cell. This is part of our history. Myth is about the body's journey, recreating itself endlessly in a particular way, to form an individual personal structure called self.[8]

Could it be that we know how to knit ourselves back together when we're broken because that knowledge is somehow an intrinsic, cellular-level property of being a body? Life can feel chaotic, meaningless, and directionless. Often it seems there's not a whiff of story structure in sight. But maybe our bodies offer us some kind of organising process, a constant storying, that when held gently, can help us make sense of the chaos.

A question I have continued to return to: how can you know, and yet not know, what you've been through? The question used a narrow definition of what it is 'to know': a cerebral cognitive knowing involving linguistic thought that can be verbally communicated. But when my body in therapy, through structures of preparation, confrontation, and integration, started writing out its emotional signatures with exuberant sweeps of its pen, I started to discover a different kind of knowing. Perhaps we were born already versed in what Keleman calls the 'poetics of the body'[9] and the shape of paragraphs, sentences, and stanzas aren't so much lofty, disembodied, cerebral concepts, but expressions of our physical form.

~

There are many parts of van der Kolk's *The Body Keeps the Score* that I found moving. None so much as his account of a form of body-based psychotherapy, which, interestingly for our purposes, is known as a 'structure'.[10]

During a structure, the client would sit at the centre of a group, recruiting people or objects to represent figures from their past, placing each representative at a location in the room and entering into dialogue with them. In this way, the client is able to physically restructure their story in space and rescript past scenarios, 'as if you could go back into the movie of your life and rewrite the crucial scenes,'[11] writes van der Kolk.

He noted that clients would become so involved in the storying process that they would enter an altered state of consciousness: 'Structures promote one of the essential conditions for deep therapeutic change: a trancelike state in which multiple realities can live side by side – past and present, knowing that you're an adult, while feeling the same as you did when you were a child.'[12]

This sounds exactly like the dyadic self I've experienced

many times through altered states: old and young, scared and fearless, vulnerable and strong. Once, on MDMA, I had the sense that I was lying on my childhood bed, feeling a crushing weight on my chest. My child-self sat up and turned around and looked at me. 'I had no idea you felt so sad,' I said to her. 'You can go and play now; I'll feel this for you.' I watched as she skipped off, feeling the child-like giddiness and the grown-up heavy heartedness at the same time. Interestingly the root word of 'ecstasy' is *ecstasis*, meaning 'to stand outside oneself'. It seems the psyche can only split off and stand outside itself like this when it's held in a supportive environment, i.e. when it's safe enough to explore.

Inner maps as external structures were of great interest to Kurt Vonnegut. During an entertaining lecture that he gave on narrative, he drew various maps of stories as a series of line graphs (they're worth looking up), that rise and fall, tighten and relax like bodies.[13] Like bodies, without fail they have a beginning, a middle, and an end. At some point on Vonnegut's graphs, the clock is going to strike midnight; whatever blocks your path is going to be encountered; the Dr Robotnik to your Sonic the Hedgehog is going to appear. You are going to 'lose your identity,' as Campbell wrote, 'and enter an abyss, a nadir, the belly of the whale.'[14] The awesome terror of this confrontation may be part of the reason that we seek ways to resolve our problems without facing them, why we numb ourselves with compulsions or chemicals in an attempt to jump from act one to act three. Even though we know, because we understand stories, that it's not the way of things, that 'the only way out is through'.

If clung to too tightly, any one way of seeing recovery, including the trauma-informed way, can serve as a form of cognitive bypassing: a way of avoiding, through intellectualisation, the somatic reality of a situation (how it feels in your body right now). Ironically, psychedelics can also become a tool that people use to bypass what needs to be faced: if you're forever trying to trip your way to some kind of promised land of mental health, you're probably unconsciously avoiding something in the here and now.

This idea that I'm exploring – healing-as-storying – could serve the same futile purpose if it was used as a consistent world view. But when looked through as one of many available lenses, it has been helpful for me in interrogating what I think we're getting wrong and right in our mental health care. Part of the reason why so many treatments are ineffective, I believe, is because they fail to understand healing in the context of the body, and, you could say, because they fail to understand the body in the context of story structure. Almost all of the treatments I was offered over the years were missing at least one act in the story.

Exposure therapy, which repeatedly exposes a person to the source of their fears, shows little interest in why they're afraid, diving straight into act two's confrontation without a solid act one (preparation and resourcing). This meant that I faced the abyss, not with abandon but with resistance, leading me to dissociate during exposure exercises and misinterpret that numbing as a reduction in anxiety.

Person-centred therapy, where the emphasis is on non-judgement and compassion, was warmer in tone, with lots of reassuring elements from act one, but since it was a static encounter that ignored my body and involved only words, it kept me on the surface and prevented me from entering act two.

Psychoanalytic therapy, with its interest in the unconscious, was heavily weighted towards act three's meaning-making. But since it lacked the groundwork of act one (my therapist would stare at me stony-faced and unreactive, regardless of what I said), and the experiential confrontation of act two, the insights were seldom forthcoming. (If a therapy takes many years before the client starts to feel better, in my view, it's not working very well.)

For me, antidepressants flattened the curve of the storying process altogether. They cut me off further from my emotions and my body, meaning that the essential, shuddering terra-forming of preparation, confrontation, and integration were impossible. As long as the peaks and troughs of the story were numbed by drugs, my inner life remained an uninhab-itable planet.

Meanwhile, the most vocal critics of the medical model are very act two-y, leaning towards confrontation, focussing most of their energy on burning down the mental illness paradigm and very little on building a wholesome new para-digm for people to live in. If you deconstruct the definition of mental health problems as illnesses, then you're also decon-structing many people's definition of getting better (a reduction of symptoms). That's a serious thing to do without also doing the difficult work of reimagining what healing could mean. More on this later.

~

So many of us in the West have lost touch with the communal activities, like ceremonial dance, chanting and initiation, that can be relied upon to take the human body through story structure.

In 2023 at Breaking Convention, Europe's largest psyche-delics conference, I sat down with PhD candidate Jacqueline Anderson, who is researching trance culture in the context of ancient communal rituals. 'There are known physical and mental benefits to prolonged dancing together. It's a timeless, global thing,' she said, explaining that, while psychedelics are a fast-track route to altered states, we've never needed drugs to get high.

'I've been looking into hunter-gatherers and the purpose of their trance gatherings,' she said. 'They were great believers in initiating creativity and releasing trauma through play and fun.' She painted a picture of people communing at Stonehenge: 'They'd have had to carry everything. That's why they had musical equipment bedded into their clothing: rattles and animal teeth and such. The idea was to make as many frequencies as you could. Even though they were nomadic, they would have places where they could go and get together, including with the children, to relieve themselves of mundaneness and release energy.'[15]

Collective dance remains a central way for communities to enact timeless story structures. The kris dance in Bali depicts a battle of good and evil in which the spirit king triumphs over a malevolent force, typically portrayed as a dragon. The dancers fall so deep into the story and the rhythm that they enter altered states in which they convulse, see visions and faint. In many traditional societies around the world, such practices are particularly invaluable as rites of passage marking life stage progression. The high school prom is an anodyne echo of what initiation means: facing fear.

Story structure itself could be thought of as initiatory. In his book, *The Rites of Passage*, French folklorist Arnold van Gennep developed a framework for the archetypal pattern of change that he saw in traditional societies' initiation ceremonies. Again, it is a three-act structure: separation, transition, and reintegration. Van Gennep likened life to a house in which people move, not gradually but in abrupt bursts, over thresholds from room to room[16]. It's in these brief between-states, these liminal middle phases, (*limen* in Latin means threshold), where you are disorientated and confused, segregated from the order that defined your previous self, facing transformative chaos.

Writer Malidoma Somé wrote vividly about tribal initiation in his book, *Of Water and the Spirit*. Somé grew up in Burkina Faso in West Africa as part of the Dagara tribe. At aged 4, he was kidnapped by French Jesuit missionaries and taken to a Jesuit boarding school, where he describes physical and emotional abuse at the hands of the priests. Aged 20, he escaped to return to the Dagara, where he had to undergo an initiation ceremony, 'one of the core rituals designed to open up this magnificent world to the growing adolescent . . . where the adolescent can fit in a context, where the adolescent can see where he or she is situated in this universe.' Much like in van der Kolk's 'structure' above, a stage is set for the dramatisation of internal challenge as external challenge.

Somé describes a preparatory phase, during which the

initiates would sit around a fire, surrounded by elders who wore phosphorescent paint, causing the initiates to feel 'buried inside a huge and growing rhythmical space' and enter a trance. This burial in community was followed by a series of terrifying challenges that Somé describes as a 'journey to the underworld', including endurance in extreme heat, and a literal burial of initiates up to the neck in the earth. 'The road back to the village is through this kind of death pathway,' Somé wrote, 'any person that doesn't want to die will die. And any person that wants to die will live.'[17] (Again, in this we can draw parallels with the popularised psychotherapeutic idea that 'the only way out is through' and Carl Jung's observation that 'what you resist persists'. Most therapies will offer you some version of this maxim, but lack any ritual or enactment to enable you to embody the theory.) This transformative archetypal death of old self is followed by a homecoming of the new self who sees the world differently: 'All of a sudden, my senses were increased tenfold . . . My perceptive eyes had become so wide that I was noticing things that I normally didn't notice.'[18] Somé movingly describes walking back towards the village alongside his father and sister post-initiation, and feeling belonging for the first time.

The image that Somé leaves us with, of a person flanked by other people, is important. Through the somatic story-telling of communal rituals, traditional societies show us that your individual body is not alone: it is part of a bigger body, the body of the tribe. You need that bigger contextual body to contain your fears, to provide a safe arena in which you can rehearse them. This is what Western mental health care seems to have forgotten. I'm afraid that the trauma-informed model and medicalised psychedelics, by treating individuals with individual disorders, often forgets it too. Without these conditions of community, so much of the Western conversation about mental health seems like well-meaning busywork that obscures and overcomplicates what has always made us happy. Worse, under the banner of progress, we seem to have written off so much traditional wisdom as primitive superstition.

'If the modern world lets the indigenous world die,' wrote Somé prophetically in 1994, 'it will probably mean a long, hard trip into the future in search of the values of the past.'[19]

On this long hard trip is where we find so much research into mental health faltering: caught in an absurd topsy-turvy attempt to justify with science what we already know in our bones. Every week studies are published 'proving' that things like nature, singing, dance, exercise, and community make us happier, framing these things as prescriptions for ills rather than cornerstone characteristics of healthy lifestyles that prevent those ills.

Many of the brilliant psychiatrists and researchers I've spoken to (psychedelics researchers in particular), have said something similar to me: they feel they're using science, to borrow Amanda Feilding's metaphor, as a Trojan horse to sneak common sense past the gatekeepers. They're frustrated at having to toe the medicalised line of conservative psychiatric and neuroscientific establishments, and they feel they can't push back, since so many people's careers depend on the over-complication of distress.

Psychiatrist Professor Allen Frances used a fittingly anachronistic space travel metaphor in the *Psychiatric Times* in 2019:

We need a moon-shot mentality – and it doesn't require rocket science or new research. We have known for 50 years how to provide good care for severe mental illness. There is nothing mysterious or complicated about it. Decent housing. Easily accessible treatment. Social clubs. Vocational rehab. Positive regard, respect, and empathy. Family support.[20]

I think it was Alan Watts who said that modern society, having forgotten that it broke people down into pieces a long time ago, now sits scratching its head wondering how to put them back together. But in that head scratching, perhaps there's an opportunity for change.

Our mental health crisis almost doesn't bear thinking about. In Europe, use of antidepressants has more than doubled in the last twenty years,[21] chronic loneliness is on the rise,[22] and in 2022, the NHS reported that 18 per cent of children under 16 had a probable mental health disorder.[23] Anecdotally, if we look at our own lives, most of us probably know someone who's chronically or cyclically dissatisfied, angry or addicted. If these people are to be helped, truly and holistically, the shift needs to be paradigmatic, towards a system that focuses on preventing distress through age-old common sense wisdom. That will involve humbly walking back some of the overreaches of psychiatry and being reminded, by groups like the Dagara, of some of the central tenets of healing: how to communally witness negative emotions; how to disrupt stagnation through altered states of consciousness; how to embrace mystery without resistance; and how to engage the body's story structure.

'The state of the world today is throwing all of us into a massive initiatory experience,' writes Somé. 'We need to hold hands with one another, if we want that initiation to lead us to a homecoming.'[24]

~

I've explored a few definitions of story so far. Story as a thing with a beginning, middle, and end. Story as change. Story as a structure we inhabit. A story is also a puzzle: an eventual alignment of different pieces that reveal a picture you couldn't see before. When I landed a job as a writer on *3 Body Problem*, a sci-fi series from Netflix, I discovered an important piece of my personal puzzle: professional satisfaction. When we started shooting at the end of 2021, I understood for the first time what it meant to love your work, and what a comprehensive impact that can have on your wellbeing. I was now spending all day every day figuring out how to tell stories with emotions, gestures, words, intonation, art direction, and set design. My opinion was sought, my contribution was needed, and I was surrounded by people, all the time.

'What happened here?' asked a colleague one day on set, as she pointed at my arm. I looked down to see my sleeve had rolled up revealing the small white scars that I often forget are there.

'I used to cut myself when I was younger,' I told her.

She paused (there's always a pause). Then glanced around. No one to pass the grenade to.

'Really?' She couldn't believe it.

'Really,' I said with a reassuring smile. I didn't want her

to feel bad for asking an innocent question. Better not tell her I cut myself as recently as two years ago when *Pure* came out, or about the boatloads of psychedelics I'd been doing. Then she'd really think I was crazy.

Another silence, which I didn't fill, since the justification I would have once filled it with – 'I was seriously mentally ill' – no longer felt right, and 'I was traumatised' seems just as reductive and partial. And besides, I didn't feel I could use the past tense just yet.

We were saved by another colleague rushing over to ask me about a line of dialogue. I had to make a rewrite decision quickly, and someone else was asking about hair and make-up. It's exciting when the clock is ticking like this.

When I turned back, the colleague who'd asked about the cuts seemed to have army-rolled out of sight.

We rolled another take. The new dialogue worked. They asked me if I was happy? I said, 'I'm happy.'

'Okay we're buying that shot,' the assistant director shouted, and bodies swooped in to deconstruct cameras, lights, and sound equipment.

I crossed the set, lost in thought. You couldn't walk across the studio without stopping for five conversations and normally I loved that. But this time I peeled off behind the trailers because I wanted to be alone. I was thinking about that awkward silence and that this is how stigma usually is: silent. There was something familiar in the gap. My shame about what I did to myself. Society's confusion about what poor mental health means. People's reticence to ask about pain. My shame at having borne pain so painful it can't be asked about.

What they don't tell you about the ups and downs of getting better, is that when the 'symptoms' start to subside, you start to feel all the emotions that they were protecting you from. You have to re-experience the world through new eyes, engage with it from a less protected place. It's been quite a shock to me to discover that when you're not thinking about your obsessive thoughts all the time, there are deeper things to think about.

What I'd been thinking about a lot, and what that silence had just reminded me of, is that it really matters that people might think I was ill when I wasn't. It matters that all those years I believed that the root cause of my suffering was a problem with my brain, and that no doctor ever explained that it was far more complicated. It matters that neither I, my mother nor my brother gave informed consent for psychiatric medications that changed our lives forever. I hadn't had the energy to think about these things because I had been tactically preoccupied trying to untie the Gordian knot of OCD (that's one of its functions – preoccupation) but now things had loosened a little, I found I was drawn to bigger knots. Why has medicalised mental health been so dominant and persistent? Why is the idea of challenging it taboo? What led me to view a stigmatising disease framework as destigmatising?

My circumstances had moved on and my heart wanted to move on too, but I couldn't ignore these questions because they are permanently etched into my skin where people can see them. I felt I owed the teenager in me, and the siblings I fought with, and the mother we couldn't help, some answers.

The bear hunt

'Stumble trip!
Stumble trip!
We're going on a bear hunt.
We're going to catch a big one.'[1]

Michael Rosen, author

'When I met you in Dublin in 2017, I identified with a diagnostic label of obsessive compulsive disorder,' I said to Dr Claire Gillan on the phone in 2022. 'I was part of an advocacy movement that holds diagnosis dear. It was a consolation to me when I found out that other people have intrusive thoughts, and that they act out compulsions. But ultimately, I found it was a false consolation, and that in the long run, it didn't help me get to the heart of what was wrong. Over the past five years I've started to see my mental health through a trauma lens . . . I wonder if the diagnostic system obfuscates what's really going on for a lot of people.'

'The things we know that increase the likelihood, with the

strongest effects, of all mental health conditions, are early childhood adversities; stressors that happened to people,' Dr Gillan said. 'It's a huge area, it just maybe didn't capture people's attention the way images of brain scans did . . . I think about this an awful lot because I teach the undergrad psychiatric disorders class at Trinity, and every week it's the same story, with disorder after disorder after disorder. It becomes quite clear what the common denominator is.'

'You're finding that adverse childhood experiences are the common denominator?'

'It's not *my* finding, there's a huge literature on this. It's not deterministic. You can't take someone into a doctor's office and triage them for mental health treatment just because of adverse childhood experiences (ACEs). But it's one of the more consistent findings that there is.'

I asked her about the role of genes in mental health. Many people are of the conviction that their chronic distress must have been genetically predetermined because others in their family have mental health problems too.

'Mental health traits and personalities are so infinitely complex. You can't reduce it down,' Dr Gillan said. 'These very complex traits arise from combinations of likely thousands of genetic variants, all conferring a very small amount of risk that we're not able to map and track in the kind of sample sizes that we have. And it seems implausible that we ever will.'

I told her how hard it is to know what to believe, when public discourse about mental health is a cacophony of mic drop moments and social media spats. 'It's quite difficult as a lay person who doesn't have a scientific background to understand these debates,' I said. 'On the one hand, you have the so-called anti-psychiatrists, who emphasise social causes of distress; on the other hand, you have psychiatrists, who think that if we keep pushing with the science for long enough, we will find the biomarkers or genes that underpin diagnostic categories. What are your thoughts on that?'

'It's hard to imagine people still wedded to a vision of a biomedical future,' Dr Gillan said. 'I can't think of any serious academics who still fall down on the hard biomedical side.' She explained to me that a few decades ago, doctors and researchers were indeed convinced of the disease model. 'Since then there's been a kind of reversal in scientific circles,' she said.[2]

~

In the 1980s and '90s, there was an explosion of interest in neuroscience. Neuroimaging technology became much better. Scientists were excited that they could take pictures of people's brains. These pictures were attention-grabbing, and journalists liked writing stories about them for that reason. Psychiatrists in their turn were excited by the prospect of mental health becoming as scientifically rigorous as other fields in medicine.

In partnership with the National Institute of Mental Health (NIMH), President George Bush declared the 1990s The Decade of the Brain.[3] Billions in public money was spent on the hunt for the biological causes of mental health diagnoses. Meanwhile, the publication of the third edition of the *Diagnostic Statistical Manual of Mental Disorders* (*DSM-III*) in 1980, had greatly increased the popularity of biological

psychiatry, and there was widespread hope of finding biological evidence to support the *DSM*. The word got out to
the public about these new frontiers of science and their
potential to unlock the secrets of human distress. This excitement fed back into the research, where amid the hype, a
huge amount of professional prestige was potentially up for
grabs. The enthusiasm was understandable, as there were
positive precedents.

In 1905, for example, through an impressive series of
scientific achievements, previously inexplicable symptoms of
depression, mania, psychosis, and delirium were discovered
to be caused by a specific bacterium, *Treponema pallidum*,
aka syphilis. A treatment was developed and the symptoms
abated. This is a shared dream of so many of us with serious
mental health problems: that a single biological root cause
will be identified and a cure developed. In *Pure*, I wrote about
my 'longing for the bleeding wound or the fractured bone.
The straight-up-and-down brokenness of injury. Here it is.
Look at it. Tell me what you see. Fix it.'[4] Imagine if we had
found a biological root cause for depression, or anorexia, or
OCD, and an effective and reliable treatment pioneered as a
result. How much suffering could have been prevented?

But – and it's a big but – the hunting party came back
empty-handed. Over several decades of research, no biological explanations were uncovered, or anything that could
be meaningfully translated to the clinic to make people's lives
better. While in all other branches of medicine, scientific
discoveries were leading to great medical leaps forward, when
it came to mental suffering, there was comparatively little to
find.

But so much had been invested, so many careers built, so many ambitions stated, that the lack of findings was a hard pill to swallow. It took a long time for the industry to admit what was happening. The reversal, as Dr Gillan described it, was slow.

It was hastened by a psychiatrist and neuroscientist called Thomas Insel, one of the most prominent figures in Western mental health research in the last half-century, who was dubbed 'the nation's psychiatrist' by the *New York Times*. During his thirteen years as the head of the NIMH, he oversaw the investment of billions in brain research. But as time wore on, he became increasingly frustrated by the lack of evidence that his huge investments were turning out. During that period, which should've been a golden age for improvements in mental health, the US suicide rate went up by 33 per cent and overdose deaths tripled.[5]

In his book, *Healing: Our Path from Mental Illness to Mental Health*, Insel describes his own epiphany – the moment he could not ignore what he already knew. He was speaking at a conference about his work in mental health research, about the new frontier of stem cells, genomics, and neurotechnology. After the lecture, during the Q&A, a man stood up and told Insel the story of his 23-year-old son, who had a diagnosis of schizophrenia, had been hospitalised and made homeless, and had attempted suicide many times.

'Our house is on fire and you are talking about the chemistry of the paint,' the father said to Insel, 'what are you doing to put out this fire?'

Insel describes how he was briefly offended by the question, and that it was this reaction that guided him. It stung because he knew that this man was right. The research he'd commissioned had done little to help the millions of people living and dying with severe mental health problems.[6]

'I spent 13 years at NIMH really pushing on the neuro-science and genetics of mental disorders,' he told *WIRED* magazine, 'and when I look back on that I realize that while I think I succeeded at getting lots of really cool papers published by cool scientists at fairly large costs – I think $20 billion – I don't think we moved the needle in reducing suicide, reducing hospitalizations, improving recovery for the tens of millions of people who have mental illness.'[7]

This was not the first time psychiatry had undergone a dramatic upheaval. Over decades and centuries, the tide had turned many times. Before the Enlightenment, as van der Kolk summarises, unusual behaviours and feelings were chalked up to supernatural beliefs: God, evil spirits, sin. Then, in the nineteenth century, we started to think of distress as adaptations to the world, as 'infinitely variable expressions of intolerable feelings and relationships.'[8] Psychoanalysts' examination of distress in the context of early childhood development and unconscious drives remained popular until the mid-twentieth century, when the tides started to turn towards biological psychiatry, which recast the range of human distress as disorders that can be fixed by medical interventions. Van der Kolk again: 'Many psychiatrists were relieved and delighted to become real scientists, just like their med school classmates, who had laboratories, animal experiments, expensive equipment, and complicated diagnostic tests . . . and set aside the woolly-headed theories of philosophers like Freud and Jung . . . the cause of mental illness is now considered an aberration of the brain, a chemical imbalance.'[9]

It's here, in this last turning of the gyre, where I'd assumed we still found ourselves. But as Dr Gillan explained to me, since the poor yield of neuroscientific and genetic research in the last thirty years, there had yet been another shift in academic circles. Now researchers were increasingly abandoning the hunt for biomarkers underpinning specific diagnoses and working transdiagnostically or adiagnostically, and there was a renewed interest in the interrelationship between biology and environment.

In the formal interviews I conducted for this book, as well as in informal ones at parties and industry conferences, I was repeatedly told some version of this. That the debate about whether or not mental health problems have purely biological root causes is already anachronistic: no one was arguing about that; no one believed the 'chemical imbalance' theory any more; and that because of the lack of etiological biomarkers, mental health had moved on to what they called a 'biopsychosocial' approach, which views mental health issues as multifactorial problems, requiring research and treatment at not only the biological level, but at psychological and social levels too.

Some professionals are so convinced of the most recent shift away from biological reductionism in psychiatry, they suggest that to criticise it is to knock down a straw man. As psychiatrist Sir Robin Murray told the *Psychiatric Times*, 'Sadly, a few psychologists appear to have been stranded in a Jurassic world where they spend their energies railing against a type of psychiatry which became extinct years ago.'[10]

In July 2022, a psychiatrist called Professor Joanna Moncrieff led a study that she said proved there had never been evidence for the serotonin imbalance theory of depression.[11] According to *Rolling Stone*, psychiatrist David Hellerstein said that Moncrieff's study was met with yawns from the psychiatric community: 'In reading it, I was kinda thinking, "Wow, next she'll tackle the discrediting of the black bile theory of depression".'[12]

Unlike many academic debates, this one went mainstream, capturing the public's imagination. Watched by millions of Britons, Moncrieff presented her findings on *This Morning*. 'We haven't so far been able to pin down any biological cause for depression,' she said.

'That's really interesting,' presenter Alison Hammond replied. 'It's actually blowing my mind if I'm honest with you.'[13]

Minds were blown all over the country. If professionals had reacted with yawns, the public did not. For them, the chemical imbalance theory of depression was far from extinct. (This is hardly surprising, since, as BBC's *Panorama* found, 'despite the lack of evidence for the chemical imbalance claim, [in 2023] it remains on half all current SSRI antidepressant patient leaflets.'[14]) In social threads and comment sections, the public reacted with understandable confusion and incredulity to hear of the lack of evidence, much like I'd done when I'd first encountered arguments for de-medicalisation. As the story spread in the press that week, I received concerned messages from friends who were taking psychiatric medications that they thought were correcting a chemical imbalance. In short, this was all news to them.

As psychiatrist and United Nations Special Rapporteur, Professor Dainius Pūras[15], told the *Psychiatric Times*, 'The most worrying feature of psychiatry is that the leadership, under influence of hard-liners, tends to label those experts who blow the whistle and critically address the status quo as anti-psychiatrists.'[16] In a UN report he explained that the problem is not so much the 'global burden of mental disorders' in individuals, but the 'global burden of obstacles being produced by archaic, broken mental health systems. Those obstacles, power asymmetries . . . the dominance of the biomedical model and the biased use of knowledge, need to be addressed by changes in laws, policies and practices.'

I started to notice a difference between what clinicians and researchers were willing to say to me on record and off record. On record, some version of this: 'psychiatry is biopsychosocial, the dark days of biological reductionism are behind us'. Off record, some version of this: 'the people who pull the purse strings are still attached to the idea of a golden age of purely biological psychiatry and no one can challenge them.'

It was this gap between the public and private message that suggested there was something worth investigating there. I don't believe this gap was disingenuous or thought through, I just think a lot of mental health professionals are following scripts without realising and are not incentivised to look beyond them. I recognise this because I lived those same well-meaning scripts for years through my advocacy.

I could see how it could be argued that, theoretically, the mental health system has moved on towards a biopsychosocial approach. But theory is not the same as practice. In 2022, over 8 million people were prescribed antidepressants in England (biological interventions) while only 1.5 million people were prescribed psychological therapy (psychological interventions),[17] and as for social interventions, I couldn't find any statistics. I suspect there's very little will in politics and psychiatry to support that research and fund this important work, because the idea of things like hobbies, community engagement, and exercise being rebranded as 'social prescriptions', operationalised, and doled out like medicines represents an awkward clash of paradigms. Academic papers like the following, entitled 'Social prescribing: where is the evidence?', tie themselves in jargon knots over this clash:

Methodological problems with generating a robust evidence base are considerable. Given the fact that social prescriptions are local context dependent and necessarily heterogeneous, there is confusion about the nature of what constitutes social prescribing. Linked to this, the multiple components that constitute a social prescription mean that evaluations are likely to be difficult to manage, compare, and assess for quality.[18]

The paper concludes that 'social prescriptions have the potential to greatly benefit individuals with complex health and social care needs' while highlighting how difficult it is to define and quantify their benefits.[19] It hits the nail on the head as to why, in my opinion, the medicalisation of human grief and flourishing is so nonsensical.

I had assumed the persistence of a biomedical hard line

in psychiatry based on my experience and the experience of my loved ones, of the mental health system in practice, where the context had been explicitly and almost exclusively biomedical. Away from psychiatric journals (that few outside the profession read), and away from expensive industry conferences (that no one outside the middle class can afford to attend), a purely biomedical model is not an anachronism from the Jurassic, it's reality.

You feel like shit, anxious all the time, and can't get out of bed. The friends you've spoken to have all asked the same question: have you thought about speaking to someone? You can't afford private therapy, so you book a doctors' appointment. You sit in a waiting room next to a rack of leaflets organised by diagnosis. While you wait, you go to the bathroom and are welcomed by a sharps bin, a hazardous waste bin, and sometimes, as if you didn't feel depressed enough, a stool chart. Your name is called. You see a doctor with a medical degree on the wall and a stethoscope around their neck. Behind them is a picture of the human heart, and in the corner there's a skeleton, each bone of which is accurately labelled with a name. You tell the doctor you've been feeling like shit, anxious all the time and can't get out of bed. They may ask about your job, relationships, and sleep, but however much they may believe in a psychosocial approach, they are almost powerless to help you in these areas. What they can do is use the limited tools and biological language they've been given to assess the severity of your 'symptoms' against industry standards. After ten minutes in this unmistakably medical environment, you come away with a prescription for a medicine, and, if you're lucky, a months- or years-long waiting list place for therapy. Even then, therapy will rarely offer practical help with your circumstances, or connect you to causes bigger than yourself. It's more likely to move you through a manualised protocol designed to change the way you think about your life rather than change the things in your life that are making you unhappy. Regardless of any theoretical nuance among professionals, very few patients/clients/service users, call us what you will, have seen any evidence of a shift away from biomedical psychiatry. Even as an advocate who was more engaged in mental health issues than most people, it took a concerted effort for me to break out of the echo chamber.

'We are all bombarded with messages about "mental illness" being "as real as a broken arm", and needing to be managed by drugs "just like diabetes",' writes psychologist Lucy Johnstone. 'Even the dubious compromise that is the "biopsychosocial" model – a way of acknowledging some role for psychosocial factors while at the same time instantly relegating them to "triggers" of a disease process – is not much in evidence on the ground . . . the biomedical message is reinforced by the fact that these labels are applied by doctors and nurses, working in hospitals and clinics, who use not just the labels themselves but the whole medicalized discourse of symptom, patient, prognosis, treatment, relapse, and so on.'[20]

The problem with a compound word like biopsychosocial is that it implies a triad of approaches, each with equal weighting, as if someone embarking on their journey through the mental health industry today would be helped socially just as much as psychologically and biologically. If we wanted to weight the word so that it accurately reflected the offering of the mental health system, it might look more like this:

biobiobiobiobiobiobiobiobiobiobiobiobiobiobiobiobio-
biobiobiobiobiobiobiobiobiobiobiobiobiobiobiobiobio-
biobiobiobiobiobiobiobiobibiobiobiobiobiobiobiobbio-
biobiobiobiobiobiobiobiobiobiobiobiobiobiobiobiobio-
biobiobiobiobiobiobiobiobibiobiobiobiobiobiobiobio-
biobiobiobiobiobiobiobiobiobiobiobiobiobiobiobiobio-
biobiobiobiobiobiobiobiobiobiobiobiobiobiobiobiobio-
bioobiobiobiobiobiobiobiobiobiobiobiobiobiobiobiobio-
biobiobiobioiobiobiobiobiobiobiobioiobiobiobiobiobio-
biobiobioiobiobiobiobiobiobiobiobioiobiobiobiobiobio-
biobioiobiobiobiobiobipsychopsychpsychopsychopsychopsy-
chopsychopsychopsychopsychopsychopsychopsychosocial.

What troubled me was that mental health professionals seemed to understand that they were using 'mental illness' like a metaphor and a value judgement about how much someone's distress was affecting their life, rather than a statement of biological reality; whereas the public generally assumed that mental illness was literal. (I started asking mental health professionals to define mental illness. They variously *ummed* and *ahhed*, chuckled, or declared the question subjective or unanswerable. You can do this experiment yourself and see what comes back. Then go ask an oncologist to define cancer.)

I wanted to know what accounted for the gap in knowledge between what the mental health professionals know, and what the public knows. Was it a failure in communication? Was it that the bear hunt of the 1980s and '90s departed very loudly and, with the exception of a few renegades like Insel, came back very quietly? That would be understandable (we all publicise our celebrations more than our disappointments – while we're crawling back into the shitpipe, we tend not to post about it). Or was there more to it? Were there forces that were tacitly suppressing the emergence of a new story?

I'm generally very sceptical of grand conspiracy narratives. I do not think that nuance is strategically being concealed by cartoonish pill-pushing psychiatrists bent on promoting a biomedical worldview for profit. Regardless of where they sat on the biopsychosocial theoretical spectrum, almost everyone I spoke to was thoughtful, held common sense, good-faith positions, and, crucially, cared deeply about helping people.

But despite decades of good intentions, the mental health system is failing abysmally, and for whatever reasons, there has effectively been an historic gatekeeping of information, as if people can't be trusted with knowing how complex mental health really is. I wanted to understand that gatekeeping process, since it'd left me and my family and our whole community in the dark about what mental health problems mean.

When a powerful group has access to knowledge that another group does not, it can be called an 'epistemic injustice'.[21] It's a phrase coined by philosopher Miranda Fricker and has been used by critics of psychiatry to describe the gap between the public's assumption about the wealth of evidence for organic biological causes of mental health prob-lems, and the industry's knowledge of how little evidence truly exists.

I took these thoughts to Dr Gillan. 'It seems that there's a kind of hierarchy in terms of who knows what,' I said to her. 'You guys are ahead because you're doing the research; the healthcare system is slower to catch up; and then we have the advocacy space and sufferers themselves. And we've been the last to know that the reality is much blurrier than the story we've been sold for the past forty years about what mental "illness" is.'

'I can see that take,' she replied, 'over-medicalisation and reductionism has caused harm. But we're wrong all the time, right? So if we translate [new models] too quickly to the end user, I see that as being problematic too. People are often too keen to move quickly forward, which can cause harm. A lot of people are not comfortable with fast translations . . . I'd be interested to hear your take on whether you think it is appropriate that we communicate all the way down to the end user?'

'I think that there's little awareness of the current debates in the general population. And I do think that's a problem,' I replied. 'This idea that has been popular for a long time, that it's destigmatising to talk about mental "illness" because it relinquishes blame . . . I think it is time to start challenging that more publicly. We've been talking about how you can't think of a respectable professional that actually believes in the "illness in the brain" paradigm, but your average person on the street is not getting that message. I think we can let people know they have a little more freedom to think about their own mental health problems. You don't have to take on a diagnostic label. People take on those labels thinking that they're scientific diagnoses. I'm troubled by that.'[22]

I agree with Dr Gillan that rushing out new paradigms causes harm. That's why the necessary corrective, as I see it, is not the psychiatric establishment unveiling some big new explanatory framework (which it can't do anyway), but rather being open and very vocal about how much mystery still abounds in the science of mental health. One thing that could be said to define the history of mental health care is a paternalistic imposition of narrative rather than a facilitation of self-enquiry and independent thought. We shouldn't be rushing to replace one spoon-fed story for another. Sometimes, 'we don't know' is a hard thing to say, but when it comes to most of our questions about mental health, mind and consciousness, it's the only appropriate answer.

Whereas poetry, art, and music have forever been able to see deeply into our suffering, early twenty-first-century neuroscience and genetics currently see comparatively little. True science, and the Enlightenment values which underpin it, embraces doubt and mystery, that's part of the excitement. 'The whole culture of scepticism', says writer and philosopher Charles Foster, 'is one which admits of exuberant, wild possibilities'.[23] In his book *Being a Human*, Foster offers us a wonderful metaphor, which points to the importance of embracing complexity. The Enlightenment Age, he posits, was a *prismatic* age. 'It takes a prism to show that white light is anything but white: that it's composed of many colours'.[24] If we're to overcome our mental health crisis, we need to think prismatically. We need to resist simplifications and be inspired by the certainty that we are always doubtless missing some richer shades of complexity on the other side of the prism. In many ways, our challenge is not to demystify mental health, but to re-mystify it.

And yet there are things we can say with confidence: that in keeping with common sense, there's very strong evidence that environmental challenges significantly increase the likelihood of someone developing mental health problems; that mental health and ill health are defined differently by different cultures, and that diagnostic specificity is a construct.

When I explained to Dr Gillan that I had come to see my mental health problems less like diseases and more like maladaptive mechanisms that once protected me from pain, she offered a cautionary note. 'There are many people who have OCD that have not had trauma,' she said. 'Different people that might experience a similar kind of trauma to you might have different mental health symptoms that might be expressed differently . . . I wonder what you think about that?'

It was a great question; one that reminded me why I loved writing this book and why I was doing it – to try to clarify what I think. It stumped me and I didn't have an answer, just another question: 'How do you measure that? How do you measure whether or not someone has trauma?'

'Well, across all mental health science, you're relying on people's self-report. Studies do it in different ways. They follow people through time, or get people to recall traumas that they've had, looking backwards. But they're not perfect. And people make their mistakes of recollection. Like all science, it's complicated, because certain kinds of people may be less likely to remember traumatic events, and that can be sometimes part of resilience, or part of the trauma itself and dissociation.'[25]

Here we get to a double bind at the heart of mental health science. Given the absence of biomarkers, self-report is almost exclusively what we have to go on, and we must take self-report data seriously, since what people say about their experience is more important than what anyone else thinks. But the people who most need help might be those who've developed sophisticated defences against self-knowledge. At the same time, it would be inappropriate, hubristic, and even harmful for any professional to suggest that a patient is in denial.

If a person with a diagnosis of OCD says they don't have a trauma history, we can do nothing but believe them. Just because, for much of my life, I was burying my feelings far below where any self-report exercise could reach, does not give me the authority to assume anyone else is doing the same. And yet I'm worried that people with trauma are falling through the net because our experiences are not easily captured by words or numbers, and that apparently evidence-based treatments are failing us as a consequence.

I do think there's something problematic about the idea of trying to quantify human emotion. If you could find someone with an identical trauma history to me on paper (the same socio-economic background, a parent with a psychiatric diagnosis, violent interactions at home) who'd grown up to be mentally healthy, and you tried to account for the differences between them and me, you would still know nothing about what had happened in our hearts and the intimate complexities of our relationships. It's almost impossible to create control conditions for human beings.

After fifteen years of being analysed, assessed, and evaluated, I've come to think that there's something irreducible about what I went through, with elements that will never be grasped by me, let alone by a doctor. And that's reasonable. I can't say for sure why I've felt the way I've felt. I can't prove to any scientist or any reader that my difficult past was the biggest contributor to my mental health problems, any more than you can prove that you grieved a person you lost, or that you love who you love. Grief, love, trauma – these things are all beyond what science can currently capture and yet are also the truest things in the world. If we can live with this paradox, maybe we can live with another: mental health problems are both out of the grasp of current scientific knowledge and deeply real.

~

I called Dr Sara Tai, a professor of clinical psychology and the director of the Psychoactive Substances Research Unit at the University of Manchester. I told her that I felt like a fool for thinking for so long that I had a disease in my brain, one that was comparable to physical disease.

'That sounds very familiar,' she said. 'I hear a lot of people saying that . . . I'm not really sure what else you're expected to think or do. You're told these messages by professionals who we've been told we should trust, so of course, you're going to believe that. When people find out that perhaps that wasn't the case, they often feel stupid, or like somehow it was their fault.'

'I kind of felt like I had the wool pulled over my eyes. Like this medical paradigm is serving the mental health system better than it's serving sufferers themselves.'

'Absolutely.'

'So what is the agenda? Why does diagnosis still have such a strong hold on the whole . . . industry? I'm going to say industry because it feels like an industry.'

'It is,' she said. 'Look, I might sound overly cynical here, but I think it's a financial one. If we don't have diagnoses, then people can't be prescribed certain drugs and drug companies won't make as much money in countries like America where they pay for their health care. If you haven't got a diagnosis, you can't bill your insurer for the care that you get.'[26]

I've tried to resist any simplistic narrative about psychs' motivations in maintaining the status quo. I think many psychiatrists tend to subscribe to the biomedical model because that's just *the way things are* and have been historically, and because they can't see the water they're swimming in. It seems that we have a collective shifting baseline syndrome when it comes to medicalised psychiatry, whereby we think what's happening is normal because the shifts have been incremental and most of us can't remember it being any other way. But as we have seen, we need only skip backward seventy years (or skip forward seventy years?) to arrive at a time when psychiatry in its current guise doesn't exist. Right now, the medical model seems impossible to dismantle, having become literally codified and manualised to meet the administrative and financial needs of pharmaceutical and insurance companies, in turn ensuring that doctors are not incentivised to see the water. Altered states of consciousness are very helpful in this regard, since their disruptive nature makes the water unignorable.

One thing I struggled with back in 2017 when I first fell into these subjects, was how to even talk about mental health without using medical language. Since then, it's been heartening to learn of other knowledge systems that do just that. Many Aboriginal and Torres Strait Islanders, for example, use the term Social and Emotional Wellbeing (SEWB), which encompasses body, mind, emotions, community, culture, family, and spirituality (the SEWB diagram is worth looking up). Mental health beyond medicalisation is clearly possible, so why does it currently seem like such a remote possibility in the UK?

Dr Tai agrees with me that there are no arch baddies deliberately peddling medicalised stories for profit. Rather, she thinks, people in the psych world are caught up in a web of administrative, commercial, and cultural influences and incentives that are bigger than any one of us and hard to untangle. 'I don't think it's because they are sitting there counting the money,' she said. 'Most psychiatrists genuinely are in the job because they want to help people. And they've been taught that that's how you help people . . . We're also stuck culturally in messages where healthcare professionals know best: they're the experts. I don't agree with that, either. I think that the people I work with, they know best, they know what works for them. My job is just helping them focus . . . keeping them on target so that they can find the answers and solutions themselves. To do that means that you have to take a step back and think, "I'm not an expert." Now you're not comfortable with not being the expert, because you've been brought up and trained in medical school and told that you are the healer. How can you ever shift perspective?'[27]

I would add that if we're forever nominalising psychiatry (i.e. using that name as if it's a monolithic thing rather than a massive group of persons, each with their own agency), then it's hard to make progress. It would be naive of me to ignore the examples of careerism I saw while researching this book. Unfortunately, I believe there are researchers and clinicians, particularly in America, who refuse to speak against models which they know to be unscientific, because to do so would be professionally disadvantageous. There's a balance to be struck. While I'm keen to emphasise that no one individual is to blame for the systemic myopia in mental health care, we must keep batting the ball back into individuals' courts to find solutions. Our job as 'service users' is not to have the answers but to keep echoing the words of the man who challenged Thomas Insel and keep asking of our mental health professionals, 'What are you doing to put out this fire?'

Psychiatry and psychology are overdue an internal reckoning, not just with the power of prestige and financial bias, but with the power of stories. As much as they can facilitate healing, stories can also lead to entrenchment. As much as narrative structure can open up the world for us, it can also close us off if its bars become too rigid. Ultimately, it's the stories we fall in love with, that we cling to for salvation and share in hope or desperation, that are driving the psychiatric juggernaut. The biggest story of them all, the one with which I made a name for myself, and the one that I wanted to look more closely at, was *diagnosis*.

Diagnostic dogma

'If science addresses itself properly to its subject of real existence rather than to neurotic affirmation of its own presumptions, it will be an epic and mystical calling, for existence is epic and reality is mysterious.'[1]

Charles Foster, writer

The *Diagnostic Statistical Manual of Mental Disorders* (DSM), psychiatry's reference text for diagnosing mental health problems – known in psychiatric circles as 'The Bible' – is the ossified spine propping up the status quo in mental health.

Psychiatrist Professor Allen Frances, who was part of the taskforce that created the third edition of the DSM (*DSM-III*) in 1980, and who led the taskforce that created *DSM-IV* in 1994, is one of the leading figures in American psychiatry and also one of its fiercest critics. 'There is no definition of a mental disorder. It's bullshit. I mean, you just can't define it,' he told psychologist Gary Greenberg in 2019, 'these concepts are virtually impossible to define precisely with bright lines at the boundaries.'[2]

When I first learned of Frances's views I was incredulous. The guy who literally wrote the book on diagnosis saying that diagnosis was bullshit? This struck me as deeply significant. And yet, just like I'd never heard of Thomas Insel, I'd never heard of Allen Frances. For reasons I was curious to learn about, these voices were not bubbling up through the industry to reach the people whose lives diagnosis impacted the most.

Via a series of publications,[3] conversations, and in his book *Saving Normal*, Frances offers an insider view of how psychiatry came to be dominated by diagnostic thinking, describing the creation of *DSM-III* as chaotic, unscientific, and riven by conflicts of interests.

In a 2022 podcast, Frances recalled how the *DSM-III* taskforce leader, a charismatic psychiatrist called Bob Spitzer, assembled a team of up to fifteen psychiatrists, usually at the New York State Psychiatric Institute, and together they decided what diagnoses would be included in 'The Bible'. How did they decide? Not with biological evidence from brain scans or blood tests, since no such evidence had ever been found. Instead, by batting around ideas about what they'd seen in clinic, and arguing amongst themselves about what was and wasn't a disorder. Spitzer would type furiously while the psychiatrists hashed it out – Frances described 'a lot of screaming and yelling about this criteria, that criteria, this diagnosis should be in, that diagnosis should be out' – then everyone would vote on the final decision. According to Frances, psychiatrists would come with their 'pet diagnoses', heavily biased by desire for prestige and financial ties to the pharmaceutical industry, which they wanted to see included. Those who were the most senior and loud, or who had the closest connection to Spitzer, tended to be the ones who were successful.

In the mornings of these day-long meetings, Frances recalled, everyone would turn up raring to go. The arguments would be heated. Then Spitzer would order 'a big pastrami deli lunch, lots of pickles. And everyone would get really tired'. As a result, the afternoon's discussions would be much less animated, as, in their post-lunch lethargy, the psychs would be less motivated to scrutinise the suggestions of others or argue their own cases too strenuously. Meaning that diagnoses that went on to influence the treatment of millions of people were potentially conceived in a food coma.[4]

I want to take a step back and focus on what really matters in all of this: the pastrami. We don't know if it was breaded or peppered, but there were pickles, we know that much. And this was New York, where they take sandwich fillings seriously, so we can assume a high-quality buffet. That lethargy-inducing pastrami is a metaphor for the platter of subjective biases that shape our thoughts and feelings without us realising. Subjectivity is human, we can't escape it. But problems arise when the subjectivities of one group are systematically repackaged as objectivities.

When *DSM-III* diagnoses were exported and promoted by the American Psychiatric Association, the thoughts and feelings of a host of powerful people got written into history as fact. Meanwhile the thoughts and feelings of the people they purported to serve got written into history as disorders. This gets to the heart of the problematic leader–follower dynamics in mental health care. Patients' opinions are often assumed to be symptomatic of underlying dysfunction (illness, trauma, etc), while doctors' opinions are doled out as gospel, though they are themselves shaped by many subjective factors (training, interests, luncheon meat, etc.).

One of the reasons I'm worried about psychiatry and medicalised psychedelics joining forces in what's been called a mental health 'revolution',[5] is that in the recent history of the psychedelic renaissance, as in psychiatry, the subjectivity of certain groups (researchers, WEIRD populations) has carried far more weight than others. Distress, altered states of consciousness, and healing: these are subjective processes where fixed definitions ought to be resisted rather than codified. A psychedelic philosophy that arises out of the psych industry's penchant for modelling, analysing, labelling, and manualising, could be a house built on sand.

~

I got some funny looks in London's Wellcome Library as I muttered, fidgeted, and sighed my way through the *DSM*. I had two editions in front of me: *DSM-IV* (because it was used until 2013, and would have been the version that guided the professionals who told my mother she had bipolar disorder, my brother that he had ADHD, and led to me being prescribed antidepressants in my teens); and *DSM-V*, which scaled up the ambition of the previous edition by adding more disorders, and has been by far the most influential edition. It sold $20 million worth of copies in its first year.[6] Each edition is nearly 1,000 pages long.

I knew that the evidentiary bar for inclusion in this book had been low, arguably non-existent. I knew that while many doctors took it with a pinch of salt, the scale of its influence had been immeasurable. I knew that it had been one of the most important books of the twentieth century and one of the most widely criticised. But I wasn't prepared for the weight of this book, in all senses. To see so much variety and depth of human experience reduced to clinical language and cut up into arbitrary pieces; the sheer volume and repetitiveness of the entries; to absorb over several hours the assertiveness and credulity of its tone; to imagine the stories *not* told within its pages.

The introduction to *DSM-IV* says, 'A common misconception is that a classification of mental disorders classifies people, when actually what are being classified are disorders that people have.'[7] Straight out of the gate, the authors unwittingly call out their own epistemological error, the one at the heart of our mental health system: an assumption that 'disorders' can be decontextualised from the humans experiencing them.

What I found striking was the way that the fundamental problems with diagnosis were casually called out in the introduction as though they are minor caveats, such as:

Although this manual provides a classification of mental disorders, it must be admitted that no definition adequately specifies precise boundaries for the concept of 'mental disorder'.[8]

And:

There is no assumption that each category of mental disorder is a completely discrete entity with absolute boundaries dividing it from other mental disorders or from no mental disorders.[9]

And:

Diagnostic assessment can be especially challenging when a clinician from one ethnic or cultural group uses the *DSM-IV* Classification to evaluate an individual from a different ethnic or cultural group. A clinician who is unfamiliar with the nuances of an individual's cultural frame of reference may incorrectly judge as pathology those normal variations in behaviour, belief, or experience that are particular to the individual's culture.[10]

To recap: there's no definition of a mental disorder; there are no definable boundaries between diagnostic categories; and diagnoses are inescapably laden with cultural prejudice. Followed by 950 pages of supposedly meaningful categorisation? The book reads like a satire of itself.

It's hard to pick a favourite entry, but 'female orgasmic disorder' is up there. According to the *DSM* it was diagnosed 'based on the clinician's judgement that the woman's orgasmic capacity is less than would be reasonable for her age, sexual experience, and the adequacy of sexual stimulation she receives'. (Imagine the scene: a group of mainly male doctors, in the early '90s, discussing whether a woman's orgasmic capacity is 'normal' and whether the stimulation she receives is 'adequate'. Would love to know if they used their own skills as a yard stick.)

My finger raced down the pages of the *DSM*, tracing the invisible connection between the ink under my fingertip and the treatments meted out to me and my family. My health records reveal that I received many separate diagnoses over the years and I was curious to see the source material. As I continued reading, I started to note down the disorders for which at one point I'd met the diagnostic criteria:

Attention deficit hyperactivity disorder
Tic disorder
Major depressive disorder
Persistent depressive disorder
Substance/medication-induced depressive disorder
Separation anxiety disorder
Social anxiety disorder
Panic disorder
Generalised anxiety disorder
Obsessive compulsive disorder
Obsessive compulsive personality disorder
Body dysmorphic disorder
Substance/medication-induced obsessive compulsive and
  related disorder
Reactive attachment disorder
Post-traumatic stress disorder
Derealisation disorder
Bulimia nervosa
Binge eating disorder
Insomnia disorder

Nightmare disorder
Oppositional defiant disorder
Alcohol use disorder
Tobacco use disorder
General personality disorder
Avoidant personality disorder
Dependent personality disorder
Caffeine use disorder
Nonsuicidal self-injury
Unspecified depressive disorder

It's not that some broad categorisation isn't useful. The above list suggests that I've historically been neurotic rather than psychotic, and knowing this could help a clinician assess my harm risks. Indeed, as Allan Horwitz explains in *DSM: A History of Psychiatry's Bible*, in the 1950s and '60s 'a basic distinction between neurosis and psychosis was sufficient for prescribing purposes'.[11] There was no need for increased granularity. Yet, this too is a distinction that should be grasped lightly, since psychosis could be thought of as being on the same continuum of disintegration as neurosis. (If a bright biological line between the two exists, we haven't yet found it.) It's also worth remembering that psychosis is a culturally sanctioned construct and that experiences like hearing voices and seeing visions are not universally viewed as pathological.[12]

Neuroscientist and psychologist Lisa Feldman Barrett offers a beautiful analogy of the way the brain imposes boundaries on continua, which I think is helpful here. She says that when we draw a rainbow on paper, we draw lines of colour, even though in reality a rainbow is a continuous gradient with no lines at all – the brain creates boundary lines to construct red, yellow, green, etc. These constructs help us communicate quickly and build a shared vision of the world. But fascinatingly, different cultures draw the lines at different places of the rainbow – the point at which 'blue' becomes 'green' is different for different cultures. While Westerners have eleven colour categories, the Himba people in Namibia have five, and therefore, the 'blue' of each group is different.[13] It's a helpful reminder that so much of what we consider objective is culturally drawn. Our predictive constructs influence how we perceive reality.

There's a meaningful and easily agreed-upon difference between two colours at the reaches of the spectrum, just like there is between someone who's suicidal and someone who's mildly depressed. While it might be helpful for the sake of organisation, communication, and harm reduction to categorise such states and everything in between, we should remember that these categories could obscure understanding as much as facilitate it, and that not everyone sees them the same.

Similarly, the 'healing-as-story' idea, which I explored earlier, is merely a construct to be held with a light touch. Real life is much blurrier. I like the way that systems theorist Gregory Bateson describes life, as 'a complicated, living, partly-struggling, partly-cooperating tangle'[14]. To me, the *DSM* is an understandable but flawed attempt to deny the involvement of all of us in that strange tangle.

When reading the *DSM* entries for mental health problems like depression, panic disorder, personality disorder, etc., I didn't see a single symptom, no matter how severe, that wouldn't be an understandable human feeling or behaviour in the face of tremendously difficult circumstances. Those circumstances are tucked away on page 715 of *DSM-IV*, in a 22-page section called 'Other conditions that may be a focus of clinical attention'[15], the purpose of which is to highlight 'the scope of additional issues that may be encountered in routine clinical practice.'[16]

Among these 'additional issues' are:

Problems Related to Family Upbringing
Relationship Distress with Spouse or Intimate Partner
Uncomplicated Bereavement
Child Maltreatment and Neglect Problems
Child Psychological Abuse
Spouse or Partner Violence
Educational Problems
Occupational Problems
Housing Problems
Economic Problems
Problems Related to Crime or Interaction with the Legal
    System
Problems Related to Other Psychosocial, Personal, and
    Environmental Circumstances

The literal separation of these core sources of distress from the rest of the book speaks volumes to me about the siloisation of our mental health system. The fact they are given 22 pages out of 950 is demonstrative of the industry's focus.

A recurrent theme in Alan Watts's hundreds of hours of

lectures is the holism, collectivism, and embodied nature of Eastern traditions in comparison with the dualism, individualism, and atomisation of the West. Reading the *DSM*, I was reminded of this insight:

> As one understands the operations of a machine by analysis of its parts by separating them into their original bits, we have bitted the cosmos, and see everything going on in terms of bits. Bits of information. And we've found that this is extremely fruitful in enabling us to control what's happening . . . we reduce the infinite wiggliness of the world.[17]

Watts gives us a useful word here: 'bitting'. The *DSM* is the starkest example of the way that the psychiatric industry has bitted us, taking social, generational, and political problems that call for multidisciplinary, systemic, holistic responses, and breaking them down into bits then analysing those bits alone as specific, medical, brain-based problems.

Our obsession with taxonomy is nothing new. Since the rise of classifications of living systems in the eighteenth century, there's been a tendency to associate classification with understanding.[18] Categories sound science-y after all. But as Dr Gillan explained to me back in Dublin, a lot of modern mental health research now seems to be blurring categories rather than creating them, suggesting that many psychiatric diagnoses could be pseudo-specific.

Leading psychedelics researcher Dr Robin Carhart-Harris notes that people across diagnostic categories have many phenomena in common: psychological rigidity, repetitive negative thoughts, a feeling of being blocked off, an inability to take reassurance on board or think about problems in new ways.[19] (This is the same general picture of 'stuckness' that'd rang true for me when I'd heard David Nutt describe a version of it in 2017.)

Along with colleagues at Imperial College London, Dr Carhart-Harris developed a general model of understanding many mental health problems called *canalization*.[20] According to the canalization model, people become ever more deeply entrenched (or canalised) into grooves of thinking and feeling, an entrenchment that seems to correlate to rigid, limited, and repetitive activity in the brain. In a way, what we call mental health disorders are less about too much disorder and more about too much *order*. The image of a canal, with its single direction and its immovable deep walls, is the metaphorical antithesis of the shaken snow globe. The unpredictability, entropy, and dynamism of the latter represents the richness and novelty that psychedelics can introduce to entrenchment. The canalization model demonstrates that a departure from diagnosis and old-school psychiatry does not mean a departure from science. Any unifying theory of understanding suffering must be held gently, but the canalization model is one that doesn't break me into bits like my medical records do.

In my experience, psychedelics don't care what diagnosis you've been given. They explode it conceptually and show you what's underneath. Psychedelics researcher Stanislav Grof called psychedelics 'non-specific amplifiers'[21] because they turn up the volume on whatever is within you. Bear all of this in mind in a few years, when you start to see marketing for psychedelic therapy targeted to your 'specific' disorder.

Right now, it behoves most psychedelics researchers to work along diagnostic lines – you get a medicine approved by showing it's effective in the treatment of a specific disorder.

'I feel very pigeonholed,' Dr Sara Tai told me. 'Unless I do research that continues to support diagnostic assumptions, I can't get funding. A lot of people don't want to talk about their symptoms. They want to talk about the real things in their life. And yet, if I don't measure *symptoms* as the main outcome of a trial, I'm not allowed to do it.'

I find it ironic that rigidity and inflexibility are the hallmark problems of a mental health system that tries to help people overcome problems with rigidity and inflexibility. I said to Dr Tai that pigeonholing in research ultimately trickles down and pigeonholes people like me at a level of our identity.

'I acknowledge what you're saying,' she said. 'I feel like I have to apologise for the profession that I am a part of. I hear stories like yours all the time.'[22]

That acknowledgement meant a lot.

~

There was something I was still trying to get my head around. If there are no biomarkers to support current diagnostic categories, and the categories themselves are not homogenous, and the whole process of diagnosis is dependent on subjective self-report anyway, what does psychiatric diagnosis actually mean to doctors, and on what grounds is its use still justified?

I called consultant psychiatrist Dr Alex Curmi at the Maudsley. I'm a fan of his podcast, *The Thinking Mind*, and I wanted to get his take.

'The first thing to point out, which is important for anyone to understand when they wade into this,' he said, 'is that diagnosis in psychiatry is different from diagnosis in a lot of other medical specialties. In psychiatry, diagnoses are based on clinical presentation, not on a cause. So if someone has a tuberculosis diagnosis, it's suggestive of the symptoms – could be cough, fever, night sweats, whatever. But it also tells you the cause, which is this very specific bacterium causing this illness. So it's a much more comprehensive description of what the problem is and how the problem is manifesting in the patient. But in psychiatry, because of the lack of biomarkers, and frankly, because there's still a lot of mystery around the conditions, the diagnosis is based purely on the presentation.'

There's that word again: 'mystery'. Dr Curmi and I agreed that we like it in the context of mental health, since it's helpful to be humble about how little we know about the complexity and depth and variety of human suffering. I explained that 'mystery' is not a philosophical position that any doctor has ever taken with regards to my case. When used explanatorily, diagnosis is decidedly anti-mystery.

'Even amongst professionals,' Alex said, 'there's a lot of debate, not just about whether to diagnose but how to use it and how to think about it.'

'Can you explain why and to what extent you think diagnosis is valuable?' I asked. I was curious to hear him steelman it.

'The best way, in my opinion, to use a diagnosis is in a very limited manner: as a snapshot description of the person's problem that helps them understand that these problems tend to cluster together; that there are other people who go through the exact same problems; and that there's a range of treatments that we can explore which apply to them and [some that] don't . . . I think diagnosis can be used badly if it's . . . a total explanation of your problem; if it's static and not subject to change, and if there are simplistic causes assigned to it and simplistic treatments. That does happen unfortunately.'[23]

My former therapist, Joyce Blake, thinks similarly. She's found that for people with intrusive thoughts of a taboo nature, diagnosis offers great relief because it normalises their experiences. 'Whilst I agree that there are currently no bio-logical determinants for OCD, and I loathe diagnostic terms such as "oppositional defiant disorder" which, in effect, gag the individual, I do feel that diagnosis can be helpful. Jung's quote sits comfortably with me as a therapist: "Learn your theories as well as you can, but put them aside when you touch the miracle of the living soul".'[24]

One of the things I've asked myself many times while writing this book is whether or not I'm getting bogged down in semantics. If one doctor talks about 'diagnosis' and another about 'distress', so what? What difference does it make if we're describing the same experience? I don't think the language itself is harmful. I still sometimes describe what I went through with terms like 'illness' and 'sickness', which make sense metaphorically.

What I'm challenging is the way that diagnostic language can give mental health professionals the authority to impose an off-the-shelf meaning onto someone else's experience. On many occasions in the consulting room, I got the feeling that I was being fit into a model, and that anything I said that didn't fit the model got overlooked. Eventually, I think

I subconsciously learned to play the game and feed my therapists' and doctors' schemas back to them, telling them the information that I knew would make sense according to how *they* conceptualised my problem. Generally, the use of diagnosis extends way beyond shorthand to become a totalising framework.

There was the time in my mid-twenties when I had intensive CBT, a modality built on a 'top down' formula that negative thoughts trigger anxiety sensations in my body. Towards the end of that therapy, I'd started to notice something that challenged this. Sometimes, actually most of the time, it was as if the anxiety sensations came first. Then a thought would pop in. I tried to explain this to my therapist, but it didn't match her understanding of the mechanics of OCD, so I dismissed it.

Years later, in 2019, after meditation and MDMA put me in touch with my physical sensations in a new way, I realised what I'd been trying to describe back then, and wrote it down: 'Thoughts rush in to narrativise bodily anxiety. Content is meaningless.' I'd figured out that, all these years, my thoughts hadn't been causing anxiety: they'd been trying to put a story to an anxiety that had always been there. It was bottom up, not top down.

The following series of notes, taken between 2020 and 2021, show why this became such an important insight for me:

December 2020: There is a gap between the thunder and the lightning, the anxiety and the thought. The trauma sensation and the invented story. The pain and the language . . . A decoupling has started.

January 2021: I don't have to escape myself. That call-back mechanism that was always putting stories to my feelings – I don't need those stories any more because I don't need to escape those feelings.

March 2021: The sensation that keeps returning, that my mind puts stories to, that sensation is uncertainty. It's asking me over and over again: are you safe? Now I can tell it: you are.

July 2021: I feel able to be present with the chest sensation without buying into or panicking about the thoughts in my head.

I wonder whether I could have come to this conclusion sooner if my observations back then had rung any bells for my therapist; if my treatment hadn't been shaped by a manualised expectation of how people with the same diagnosis present; if my case had been given an open future.

There was also the time in 2020 when I'd been assessed by a brilliant psychiatrist whom I knew personally, at one of the country's leading centres for anxiety disorders. I qualified for a twenty-week course of CBT and was put on a year-long waiting list. By the time my slot rolled around, I'd already been working separately with Joyce for some time and was making progress. CBT felt like it would be a step backwards and I almost turned the course down. But anyone who's been through multiple therapies will know the little voice that says 'maybe this time will be different'. The therapy was free and I was still desperate to heal. I figured beggars can't be choosers.

At the start of the course, my problem was conceptualised as two comorbid conditions: OCD and body dysmorphic disorder (BDD). By then I'd been working with MDMA for two years and had developed a more integrated view of my suffering as a cohesive response to stress. I no longer saw any meaningful distinction between OCD and BDD. Rather, I felt they were related attempts to solve the same problem, and that to separate them would be to miss the common source of pain that was upstream of both. My therapist (a very smart, empathetic, and skilled person whom I liked a lot) listened and understood, and did the best she could to integrate two distinct manualised treatments, one for OCD, one for BDD, but the rigidity of the system was clear. She had little room for manoeuvrability and had to use protocols which didn't lend themselves well to being blended.

Meanwhile, there wasn't space for my working theory that my OCD/BDD had, on some level, tried to protect me from pain. My therapist was concerned that this would indulge my disorders, giving them more legitimacy than they deserved. When she encouraged me to think of my OCD as a bully rather than a protector, I pushed back. I said I now thought my OCD represented the most hurt, vulnerable, and hard-working part of me and I didn't want to vilify that part any more. My therapist didn't think there was evidence that this way of seeing was helping me, and I was sent away with homework; tasked to write down evidence for two claims:

A) OCD is a bully.
B) OCD is a protector.

It makes me feel tense writing this now, to think of how many exercises like this I had to do over the years, how many boxes I'd literally ticked to show my willingness and coop- eration, to think how often I acquiesced to therapists' interpretations just so that we could move on. Having found through MDMA a map of my internal world that made sense for the first time, it was confusing to have to now redraw the boundary lines I thought I'd eroded.

That same year, as part of the research for this book, I decided to try ketamine-assisted psychotherapy, which is legal in the UK. I'd done ket at parties but never in a therapeutic setting. I paid a £360 hourly rate to see a psychiatrist who I'd been told was making referrals to an NHS-subsidised ketamine therapy clinic.

The psychiatrist's office was in Knightsbridge, the waiting- room more plush than your average. Among the old copies of *Tatler* and *Hello!*, a glossy magazine caught my eye. If my writing team was discussing ways to communicate visually how far removed from ordinary people's lives psychiatry and psychedelics had become, and someone suggested putting a copy of *Rich List* on a waiting room coffee table, I'd say it was a little on the nose. Yet there I was, calming my anxiety with tales of pork billionaires, pet kibble giants, tycoons of fasteners and slurry, and, more cheerily, Mr Ferrero's very well-earned Nutella fortune.

At the end of my forty-minute assessment, the psychiatrist leafed through his notes. What I'd reported was a mixture of symptoms and moods, sometimes anxious, sometimes depressed, and this was a problem, since I officially inhab- ited two diagnostic categories (OCD and depression) and ketamine therapy had only been approved for depression. He wanted to help me and he thought that ketamine therapy could indeed help, but he could only refer according to strict diagnostic codes.

I could feel the energy draining from me. Acceding to gatekeepers for a couple of decades tends to drain your energy. I was starting to wonder if there were any professionals out there whose hands weren't tied, who felt they could act freely on their common sense and expertise. How much hand-tying would it take before the industry was prepared to challenge the status quo from within?

The solution we came to was a farce. I was to fill out two questionnaires, one as if I had OCD symptoms all of the time, one as if I had depressive symptoms all of the time. Whichever matched more closely to the clinic's diagnostic criteria would be the one we sent. We sent the 'depressed' one, which got me a place at the clinic.

The ket clinic then sent me a link to 'an automated self-management system' called True Colours, through which I had to fill out further questionnaires twice a day for several weeks. Once enough data had been gathered, I would then go to the clinic, where I would lie alone on a hospital ward, overseen by a nurse, put on a ketamine drip, and separated by a curtain from other people also having infusions. It was a vision of biomedical psychedelics that left me cold.

When my new bestie True Colours started pinging me with friendly reminders to fill out the forms, I felt my body say 'no'. No more hoop jumping. No more using my intimate data to game the system. No more subjugating my insights to psychiatric apologists. I'd had enough. I finally put my finger on what I'd felt for a long time: that the system was not helping me. It confused me in subtle ways and challenged my agency to formulate my own story, meanwhile offering none of the non-transactional human connections, purpose or self-expression which I'd come to understand as fundamental conduits to healing.

~

I was curious to learn more about models for mental health care that didn't rely on diagnosis, so I spoke to healer Euphrasia Nyaki, the founder of a holistic centre for women in João Pessoa, Brazil. Efu, as she likes to be called, integrates traditional healing approaches from Tanzania with a wide range of practices, from somatic experiencing, to massage and reiki, herbal medicine and family constellations therapy. She explained that many of the women she treats have previously been to psychiatric hospital, where they've been diagnosed with what are culturally thought of as 'women's problems' – depression and hysteria – and have been heavily medicated. How is Efu's clinic different?

'First of all, I create the space,' she said. 'I check in with myself, to know that I don't have any defences or worries. I'm just totally relaxed. When I welcome the women in, I give them freedom to look around slowly, to connect with everybody . . . We make them juice, a very nice juice that has beetroot and carrots and greens. The women feel at home. Many comment on how just the welcome itself is already healing.'

It struck me that Efu hadn't yet mentioned anything I would previously have thought of as 'treatment'. I reflected on my own psychotherapy with Joyce. I'd never stopped to notice that the healing had begun in the way she opened the door, said 'hello', and offered me water, and had continued in the way she postured her body and mirrored my face as I spoke. We're conditioned as 'patients' to think about therapy as an intervention rather than an experience; as technical rather than relational; as an input of theories designed to achieve a specific output.

Efu continued, 'Maybe we put them into the mud therapy room. We put a little bit of mud on their face to help them relax,' she said. 'After I help them feel safe, I ask how they feel in their body. We don't diagnose the women. We ask them what is missing. We talk about their problem, a little of the story of what happened, but we don't interpret the story, we keep going back to the body, then they begin to release.' Efu described how, with no need for a diagnosis of any kind, through a repeated mindful return to bodily sensations, the women's bodies would start to shake or groan with emotion as they moved from contracted to expanded states.

There's technical skill in the somatic experiencing protocol that Efu described that can, to some extent, be manualised. But she is also showing the value of something less tangible and equally important, something that Western medicine might dismiss as soft or unscientific: an ineffable connection of safety between two people, an interplay between their nervous systems. She invokes images of home, and checks in with her own body to see if she has the capacity to be helpful. The therapy is nestled in the context of human interaction and sensory exploration (the fruit juice, the mud, the time to greet people and chat on arrival), from which it cannot be divorced.

The boundaries between therapy and life also seemed to be blurred. Efu described the centre as more like a community hub, with people coming and going at leisure, than a doctor's surgery. She explained that, back in Tanzania, there was no therapy as we'd recognise it.

I told her about Mom's hospitalisations and how they'd affected me.

'In Tanzania, everything is so communal,' she said. 'If my mother was taken away, my aunts and grandmother would take over. My grandma used to live like right next door . . . Mama is the only mama, there are no two mamas. But at least you would have some kind of resource to help you cope. So that's a very big difference from the Western culture to the indigenous communal culture where the kids are raised by everybody. When one has a problem, the others jump in.'

Efu described extended family and ancestry as inseparable from concepts of wellbeing. She thinks that part of the reason Westerners feel so disconnected from their bodies is that our connection to the bodies of our ancestors is missing.

'How can I connect with my ancestors that have passed away?' I asked Efu.

'Well, Rose, when you look in the mirror, what do you see?' She left a silence for the question to land.

It surprised me. I choked up. 'I see my face.'

'You see your face. Yes. You see your face. So, one eye for sure looks like your mother, and the other looks like your father.' She pointed playfully to each of my ears. 'Over here looks like your grandfather and over here looks like your grandmother.'

I touched my ears and laughed. Tears rolled down my face.

'How do I connect with my ancestors?' she said. 'I look in the mirror. I see myself and I know they are here. They exist because I exist. They died already. But they are alive inside of my body.'

I told her that I knew fragments of my ancestors' stories. How Papy André had slipped past his Nazi gatekeepers; how Grandma Betty had been forced to give up her baby. How I'm a secular atheist who doesn't pray. How I wanted to connect with Betty, but I didn't know how, since she never knew I existed.

'She knows,' Efu said, leaving another silence. 'Just connect to the idea that she knows.'

~

'That's all, thanks,' I said as I put the olive oil and the pack of coffee on the counter. Mindlessly, I reached for my wallet and then unfolded a shopping bag. I wasn't really there. I was daydreaming, taken off by the berries and chocolate smell of the coffee and floating belly-up, like an otter, in a Guatemalan lagoon. Within the next four weeks I had to turn half a book into a whole book, finish a feature film script and start the *3 Body Problem* writers' room for season two. Recently my body had started laying down a spike strip at night – insomnia – in an attempt to slow me down, but with flat tyres I was rolling on. I swayed gently in ripples of coffee as vanilla pods fell from the overhanging trees—

'Is it Rose?' someone said.

I surfaced and realised that the girl behind the till was looking at me. She was in her mid-twenties.

'Yes.'

She broke out into a smile. 'You're the reason I got a diagnosis of OCD,' she said.

I felt the *whomp* of emotion light up the air between us.

'Your article really helped me. And yeah' – she faltered – 'I just wanted to say thank you'.

I shook off just enough emotion to speak. 'That means a lot, thank you for telling me that.'

'Do you need a bag?' she said.

'I'm good, thanks.'

There was a sweet lull as I gathered my things. We stepped on each other's goodbyes, then I was back out on the street.

The occasions that I get stopped like this give me an opportunity to reflect on the impact of putting a story out in the world and the extent to which my understanding of mental health has shifted since writing *Pure*.

As I walked across the park (quickly, because I needed coffee and this book wasn't going to write itself), I reflected that there's a baby in the bathwater of the medical model. There's so much good stuff in the reassurance that diagnosis offers: you're not alone; others feel this way; these experiences are well-documented; you can get better. The challenge in the future of mental healthcare will be retaining that assurance while loosening the grip of the stories that initially forged it. Somehow, slowly, carefully, we've got to get the tablecloth off without breaking the glasses. Or maybe we've got to trust that people aren't nearly so fragile as we think.

I called Dr Gabor Maté, one of the most vocal critics of the status quo in health care, for his advice. I was conscious of the grey area between healthy scepticism and the new breed of blanket contrarianism on which public figures can now so easily build their careers. Vague anti-establishment, anti-industrial complex, anti-Western medicine suspicion is its own kind of tedious zealotry. At all costs I wanted to avoid any alignment with that kind of dogmatism by being as careful and precise as possible. I knew that my new book would dismantle some of the comforts of the old one and I wanted to do that delicately.

Rose: I want to challenge the dominant paradigm but I'm also aware of how attached many fellow sufferers are to this notion that they have an illness. I was wondering if you had any advice about how I can bring that critique without shattering anyone's world view or upsetting anyone too much.

Gabor: But you have to shatter people's world view. They have a false world view. If you had a false world view, would you want to hold on to it, or to have it revealed as false? What would you like?

Rose: Of course, I would rather have it revealed as false.

Gabor: So what's your concern?

Rose: I think part of the reason why I was so drawn to the idea that I had a biological disorder in my brain was that it was a story, and I think we need stories—

Gabor: Well, you did have a biological disorder in your brain, that's not the point. The point is, where did that biological disorder come from? Let me just go through a few steps if that's okay? You said a diagnosis of OCD explained your problems?

Rose: That's how I felt at the time, yes.

Gabor: No it didn't, it explained nothing. How did you know that you had OCD?

Rose: I was having repetitive intrusive thoughts and I was acting out mental compulsions.

Gabor: Why were you having repetitive intrusive thoughts and acting out mental compulsions?

Rose: Because I had OCD.

Gabor: How did you know you had OCD?

Rose: I see.

Gabor: You've explained nothing. Psychiatry confuses descriptions with explanations . . . I've been diagnosed with ADHD, because I have difficulty with focussing and sitting still and impulse control. Why do I have difficulty with focussing and sitting still and impulse control? Because I have ADHD. It's bullshit. It's totally tautological. So diagnoses can be useful descriptions, but they don't explain anything. The explanation is that your compulsive thoughts are actually an escape from much more painful emotional dynamics and memories that you weren't ready to deal with . . . Everything is biological. Walking, eating, thinking, dreaming. The question is where does this biology come from?

Now the mainstream explanation is that it is genetically determined, for which there's zero evidence. Nothing. Zilch . . . There's some genetic input, which I can talk about, but no mental disease is determined genetically. Nobody's ever found a single gene, or a group of genes, that if you have it, you'll have a certain mental disorder. And if you don't have it, you won't.

Gabor went on to explain that, having reviewed all of the available literature on genetics and mental health while researching his latest book, *The Myth of Normal,* he'd concluded that what's been proven is that some people have a genetic predisposition to sensitivity. This sensitivity could increase a person's vulnerability to developing mental health problems, if (and only if) they're exposed to stressors. But sensitivity does not equate to mental ill health.[25]

There's a metaphor that might be relevant here, proffered by a 2005 paper on child development: some people are orchids, some people are dandelions. Some are highly sensitive to their environments, some will flourish in adverse conditions.[26] Though it's a binary and simplistic image, I like its redemptive reminder that none of us are predetermined to wither; all of us have the capacity to thrive.

Rose: I think a lot of doctors know that it's bullshit and they know that they're using diagnoses as constructs, whereas people receive them as [literal explanations] . . . I would love to hear your thoughts about what accounts for that gap.

Gabor: First of all, I'm not so sure that doctors are that aware that it's a construct. Nothing in my education prepared me to understand that, and I don't see much in the education of doctors now. I really do think doctors see diagnoses as explanations . . . In my days of biological determinism, people would come to me and I'd say, 'Look, you've got a lack of serotonin in your brain, and I'm gonna give you a medication that's going to improve your mood.' I spoke that way. And I was a pretty savvy GP. I was interested in mental health issues and so on . . . I'm not sure that I agree that there is a gap between what doctors understand and what the public understands. But if there is, who's responsible for that gap? All those years, when you were told that you had a biological disorder, did anybody ever tell you that your brain is actually shaped by the environment?

Rose: No.

Gabor: That's what the science has shown for decades now.

Rose: Yeah, it's not controversial.

Gabor: It's not controversial.

Rose: I'm a writer, so my interest is in story structure. I've noticed that MDMA and psilocybin experiences seem to have their own innate unfolding structure, almost like a story.

They [have] this preparation phase, this confrontation phase, and this integration phase, and it made me wonder whether the mystery of how we heal is also the mystery of how we understand stories? We're never taught to do either . . . Carl Rogers wrote about 'the directional tendency', Stanislav Grof talked about holotropism – moving towards wholeness. Both of those things, to me, mean story.

Gabor: There's always a story there. And the question is, how congruent is the story with reality? Some stories serve a function of shielding you from all kinds of pain at a time when you cannot handle it. But if the story clashes with reality, we suffer eventually. Healing is all about getting our story more and more congruent with reality.

Rose: That's integration.

Gabor: Integration, yeah. In terms of something you said earlier about disease being something that we *have*. Like, 'I have OCD' or 'I have ADHD'. That assumes that there's an entity called OCD, which has got its own characteristics and behaves in a certain way, independent of me . . . It's not true. Actually, the disorder is a process that occurs inside the nervous system, and the nervous system is in interaction with the whole world, in concentric circles, beginning with mother, and the womb, and then the family of origin and the multigenerational family and the community, and all society, and so on . . . The reason I might *have* ADHD or you might *have* OCD is because at some point I had to disconnect from myself, a defence mechanism at a time when to be fully present was way too painful. And therefore, healing has to do with reconnecting, which means wholeness. Instead of being disconnected from ourselves, we reintegrate parts of ourselves that were too uncomfortable to experience before.

Rose: Do you think the reason that the reductive biological paradigm has stuck around for so long is because we want to avoid pain?

Gabor: Well that's a big part of it. *You* know what it's like to actually realise that difficult stuff happened to you. That's painful stuff. And it also feels so disloyal to your family because, after all, *my parents loved me and they did their best.* It creates real tension for people. But there are some powerful institutional reasons why the biological framework is so dominant. It's just a lot easier for doctors. If you come to me, it'll take me five minutes to make the OCD diagnosis. Then another five minutes to prescribe the medication. But to actually talk to you about what happened to you? That takes time, not just expertise, and a kind of emotional presence.

Rose: It strikes me that the medical model is serving poor people and marginalised groups the least, because they're the people who don't necessarily need psychiatric interventions but social interventions; they need help improving their lives . . . I'm really troubled that we're telling people who've got genuinely difficult lives that the problem is inside their brain rather than outside in the world.

Gabor: Well look at Canada. I was just four days ago in Northern British Columbia, at a conference on rates of addiction, suicide, overdose, and ADHD in our indigenous population. It's just scandalously high. And it's because of historical trauma imposed by colonialism and the very deliberate destruction of their family structures, the abduction by the state and church of their children into residential schools where they were sexually, physically, and emotionally abused. It's just so clear. There was an article in the *New York Times* a few weeks ago, about how in Britain, in areas where there have been austerity cuts to youth centres, there's been a rise in youth violence.[27] What a surprise. It's poor kids and kids of colour who are most likely to be diagnosed and medicated, statistically. This is trying to deal pharmacologically with what is essentially a social problem, a structural problem in our society.[28]

I later reflected that it's not either/or. Psychiatric medication can theoretically be used in conjunction with broader social changes, but as we've seen, this integrated approach is rarely put into practice. Psych drugs can be a life-saving intervention, and psychiatry can play a vital role as a limited, risk management service, triaging people at the point of crisis. But this generally isn't how psychiatry is seen or, in my opinion, wants to be seen.

If we lionise psychiatry and psychotherapy as complete responses rather than small parts of a broader systemic response, I believe these disciplines can serve to support a deeply conservative system by helping people adjust to the miseries of consumerist society. If they are unwilling to admit that their role in healing can ultimately only ever be a modest one, I'm of the view that psychiatry and psychotherapy are only ever going to be reactionary institutions, prompting people to make psychological accommodations for the sickness in the world rather than addressing that sickness at its root.

INT. THERAPIST'S OFFICE - DAY

In a room lined with psychology books, there's a couch and two chairs facing each other. Rose sits in one of them. There's a knock on the door.

                    ROSE
          Come in.

Barry enters. Rose looks confused.

                    ROSE
          Aren't you Barry from the post
          room?

                    BARRY
          I'm a tool in your imagination.
          You tell me.

                    ROSE
          Right, yeah.

She gestures for him to sit.

                    ROSE
          Okay. So. I'm going to play your
          therapist and you're going to play
          The Mental Health System.

Barry sits. He looks unimpressed.

                    BARRY
          "The Mental Health System"?

                    ROSE
          What?

                    BARRY
          Seems a little reductive.

                    ROSE
          How so?

                    BARRY
          Reducing a complex system down to
          a single label.

A beat as they stare at each other.

                    ROSE
          Shall we start?

Barry shrugs. Rose clears her throat. Then:

                    THERAPIST
          What brought you to therapy?

The Mental Health System sighs. *Where to start?*

                         THE MENTAL HEALTH SYSTEM
                    I'm a mess. I'm all over the
                    place. I don't know who I am.

He falters. The Therapist lets him continue. The
conversation is spacious.

                         THE MENTAL HEALTH SYSTEM
                    I've been working really hard
                    for a really long time to
                    makes things better. But I'm
                    failing.

                    THERAPIST
          You've done lots of wonderful things,
          don't you think?

                         THE MENTAL HEALTH SYSTEM
                    I'd call the mental health
                    crisis a pretty big failure.

                    THERAPIST
          What advice would you give to
          a friend who said they were
          a failure?

                         THE MENTAL HEALTH SYSTEM
                    Depends how much of a fuck up
                    they were.

They laugh.

                         THE MENTAL HEALTH SYSTEM
                    I used to be so excited. I
                    really believed I could explain
                    suffering with science.I wanted
                    to help people.

                    THERAPIST
          You're compassionate. That's
          an important quality.

                         THE MENTAL HEALTH SYSTEM
                    It wasn't enough though was
                    it? I've explained almost
                    nothing.

                         THERAPIST
          How does that make you feel?

                         THE MENTAL HEALTH SYSTEM
          Embarrassed. Frustrated. Mainly numb.
          Shutting it all out.

                         THERAPIST
          We all have coping mechanisms.

                         THE MENTAL HEALTH SYSTEM
          I feel like my story is stuck,
          y'know? ts because that's all I
          can do. They say if you keep doing
          the same thing over and over with
          the same results, it's a sign of
          madness.

He laughs sardonically.

                         THE MENTAL HEALTH SYSTEM
          And I'm the one who's supposed
          to be making people <u>not</u> mad.

                         THERAPIST
          Why do you think your story is stuck?

Barry takes a sip of water.

                         THE MENTAL HEALTH SYSTEM
          Because I'm refusing to confront
          my reality.

                         THERAPIST
          What's the worst that would happen
          if you confronted that reality?

                         THE MENTAL HEALTH SYSTEM
          I could lose my job, my prestige,
          the sense of authority that I've
          got quite attached to.

                         THERAPIST
          That's understandable. Fear of loss
          is a very human thing.

There's a knock at the door. A 60-something woman in a
suit pokes her head in. She sees she's interrupting.

                         WOMAN
          Oh, sorry.

                    THERAPIST
              (smiling)
         We'll just be a couple more minutes.

The woman backs out and closes the door. The
session resumes.

                    THE MENTAL HEALTH SYSTEM
         Was that The Government?

The Therapist smiles apologetically.

                    THE MENTAL HEALTH SYSTEM
         The Government is one of your
         clients? Wheel the couch out for
         her. Fucking hell, I thought I had
         problems.

                    THERAPIST
         Sorry for the interruption. We do
         have a little more time.

                    THE MENTAL HEALTH SYSTEM
              (miserably)
         Yay.

                    THERAPIST
         What's the reality that you're
         unwilling to confront?

The Mental Health System looks into his lap.

                    THE MENTAL HEALTH SYSTEM
         If I was actually honest with
         myself about what's at the heart of
         our mental health crisis, I'd have
         to admit that I can't really help
         because it's not primarily a health
         problem, which would mean it's not
         my job to solve it.

He points to the door.

                    THE MENTAL HEALTH SYSTEM
         It's *her* job. It's everyone's job.
         It's about the way we live and the
         way we connect, and I don't have
         the answers to that stuff.

                    THERAPIST
         Isn't it okay not to have the
         answers?

Out on The Mental Health System, contemplating.

PART THREE

Integration

Nonlinearity

'Life itself means to separate and to be reunited, to change form and condition, to die and to be reborn. It is to act and to cease, to wait and to rest, and then to begin acting again, but in a different way. And there are always new thresholds to cross.'[1]

Arnold van Gennep, folklorist

The question I asked Joyce, my psychotherapist, in the autumn of 2021 is the question that all of us with chronic mental health problems are asking at bottom: 'does it ever end?'

A lot had shifted that year. I'd had three MDMA sessions with Rachel and Jonathan, several craniosacral sessions, and lots of EMDR. I'd integrated the material from these various altered states through regular meditation, yoga, and psychotherapy, and I was putting it all into practice through increasingly authentic-feeling connections with the people I love.

Earlier that year I'd had my first glimmer. The opposite of a flashback, a glimmer is a moment of calmness and presence shining through. I'd been at my brother's house with three generations of my family. The kind of gathering that my mind would've once carpet-bombed with intrusive thoughts. I noticed how soothing it was to hear so many voices layered over each other, almost humming, and how I'd never noticed this before. My little niece looked at me. I pulled a silly face and she pulled the same face back, and we both burst out laughing. Moments like that, of emotional throw and catch, had shown me that the world involved me, and that things could be different . . .

Yet months later, there I was, sobbing and bewildered in front of my therapist, feeling like I was back to square one and not understanding why.

I used to think I had a map for getting better: that one day the symptoms of my illness would subside like the runny nose of a cold. What I was learning the hard way is that getting better is not just a reduction in symptoms, it's a radical and general reorganisation of a system – a rigid and deeply bedded-in system of psychological and somatic processes. As the system reorganises, you have to slowly relearn the world without your old protections, and that's hard.

'I can't believe I'm here again,' I said to Joyce.

'It's a bumpy road,' she said, reassuring me that the person sitting in front of her today seemed remarkably calmer and more secure than the person she'd first met two years before. 'Things can get worse before they get better but I do think you're making progress.'

It was hard for me to believe her on days like that, when I could see all the single steps backwards but none of the apparent steps forwards. I'd spent the last twenty years trying to improve, and nothing had worked in the long term. My adult life had been a game of existential ping pong, of trusting in this or that modality; of finding that the powerful placebo of my belief had not been enough; of realising that the treatments that had apparently been so successful for others had ultimately failed for me. Even the MDMA therapy, which I thought was going to save me, didn't seem to be moving the dial.

The 'healing journey' metaphor implies a forward motion towards a destination. But maybe the journey is unending, maybe there is no destination, and maybe you're walking a maze. It's difficult to see clearly when you're in the dark of nonlinearity. The sharp turns obstruct your view of the exit and block its light, if you're able to keep the faith that there even is an exit. When you take a step, how can you tell which way you're facing? It helps to have a skilled therapist to hold your hand and describe the world that you can't see, but how do you know if you're pointed in the direction of resolution?

My 2021 notebook reveals the volatility of that period:

20 Feb 2021: I think this might be it. After all the years. Just had a couple of days where I had zero intrusive thoughts.

26 March 2021: 4 great days. 2 bad days. Nightmares, anxiety.

4 April 2021: Everything is going to be okay.

19 June 2021: OCD felt real. Horrific. Every time I get close to feeling anger, my OCD closes in. After several hellish days I shut down . . . walking slowly, sluggish, lethargic.

12 July 2021: The worst my OCD has ever been. How can this be real?

18 July 2021: 5 days amazing. 7 days terrible. 3 days amazing.

29 July 2021: 3 bad days. Shorter than recent stretches. Followed by 13 days of massively reduced intrusive thoughts.

Reading my notes back, I could see that Joyce had been right – the bad patches were getting shorter. Yet, when each patch came, it felt solid, absolute, and permanent, admitting no knowledge of having felt any other way, and was expressible only in superlative, black and white language. All good or all bad. I got curious about the fact that no matter how much progress I'd made, knowledge of that progress could suddenly become blocked off. I wondered if this oscillation between mutually exclusive states of emotional intensity and emotional numbing held a clue that might help me draw a map for getting better.

It wasn't a random pattern, there was a cycle of causal relationships between each state. As I wrote in October 2021:

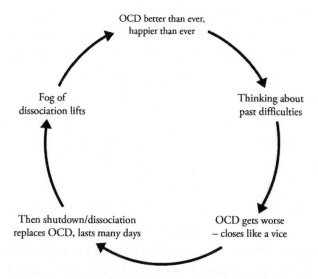

When emotions got too much, OCD would rush in as a distraction, replacing feelings related to the past with irrational preoccupations in the present: 'look over there'. Soon, the anxiety would become untenable, and I would numb out for a few days, before the fog started to clear and I'd feel well again.

I started to conceptualise the process as one of expansion and contraction, which resonated more than the psychiatric model of relapses and recoveries. As my system was gradually building the confidence to feel more intense and complex feelings (expansion), my defences were reacting in kind, intensifying in an attempt to contain a potentially threatening influx of emotion (contraction). What was difficult to notice in the moment was that each time I expanded a little more and contracted a little less. Each time I got back, as Bootsy said, to 'the one', I was staying a little longer. While the phenomenology week to week was chaos, on a bigger time scale, there did seem to be a positive directional progression in the nonlinearity.

I noticed expansion–contraction metaphors popping up across different schools of thought. Psychiatrist Dan Siegel writes of our 'window of tolerance'[2] getting bigger and smaller. Complex trauma expert Deb Dana writes of a ladder[3] that we ascend and descend. The polyvagal theory evokes the language of accelerator and decelerator pedals being alternately pressed[4]. Traumatologist Peter Levine evokes the language of a pendulum swinging.[5]

An unassuming woman I met on retreat said it best. Our group was gathered in an old library to share observations about our practice. When it came to her, she apologised and said she was nervous. Her hands were shaking, and she looked down at her lap as she described something she'd experienced while meditating that morning (the line breaks reflect her pauses):

> I was feeling resistance, resistance, resistance.
> Then suddenly I arrived at this place of no resistance –
> a huge still space where I could breathe.
> And then a thin veil of fear closed in around me.
> And I felt I couldn't go any further.

Tears filled my eyes. Others in the group felt it too; some looked down at their own laps. I suspect they felt as I did, that this woman had just ever so gently smashed through their skulls. She'd described a dynamic I'd been grappling with in my healing but hadn't ever fully expressed. The dizziness of being on the threshold; wanting to heal but fearing it. A bodily sense that if I relaxed, I would suddenly fall off a cliff. Wasn't she bang on? At the first inkling of non-resistance, wasn't that exactly when resistance reared its head? Feelings of spaciousness in my body would often constrict and solidify when I brought my focus to them. Openness and fear of openness were in constant relationship.

Throughout 2021, my body was continuing to dramatise this oscillation with a somatic nightmare: a lateral tugging from one side of my chest to the other that woke me up with a racing heart. My mind projected it as a series of psychological contradictions: I crave intimacy, but I fear it. I'm exhausted, but I'm restless. I want to leave, but I want to stay. I know it's true, but I don't know it's true.

Psychiatrist R. D. Laing gave voice to these psychological impasses in a book of creative writing called *Knots*:

> I am frightened to be frightened when you
> tell me I ought not to feel frightened.
>
> frightened
> frightened to be frightened
> not frightened to be frightened
>
> not frightened
> frightened not to be frightened
> not frightened to be not frightened.[6]

The infuriating repetition and solipsism speaks volumes to me about the kinds of dense, contracted states of irrationality, which bafflingly, despite all of my work, I was continuing to periodically plunge back into. The knot metaphor is brilliant because, just as knots get tighter when you pull in opposite directions, so too does the tangled psyche. How can you crave closeness and reject it at the same time? This seemed like an unfathomable paradox until Joyce shared with me an illumination from British psychoanalyst Donald Winnicott. He said that while a troubled child is longing to communicate, at the same time they are establishing a 'private self that is not communicating . . . It is a sophisticated game of hide-and-seek in which it is joy to be hidden but disaster not to be found.'[7]

According to systems theory, the volatility of my mental states might have been the very thing that led to opportunities for change, since instability in natural systems can create dramatic growth spurts. As one paper explains:

> In post-traumatic growth, life transition, and psychotherapy, destabilization often occurs in the context of emotional arousal which, when accompanied by emotional processing and meaning-making, seems to contribute to better outcomes . . . There is then an oscillation between old patterns that are less viable and new patterns that are emerging, until the system settles into a new dynamically stable state and variability decreases.[8]

An oscillation between old stuck patterns and disruptive new ones. This rang very true with me. I have previously described my *symptoms* as disruptors, characterising cutting and purging as attempts to break through the maddening stasis of trauma and get things moving again. Does it make sense to call both my symptoms, and my post-traumatic growth, disruptive? I think so, if we see two steps forward, one step back as the struggle to replace unhealthy disruptors with healthier ones; unhealthy ways of feeling alive with healthy ways of feeling alive.

But how could I make it end? And why was it taking so long? Looking back, it's obvious. We spent a lot of 2021 in Covid lockdowns. I was single and lived alone, and went for months without being touched by or touching another person. And even though I was gradually starting to understand that my lows were part of a directional process, it didn't make them any easier. It was little comfort to understand that nonlinearity was a feature, not a bug, of deep psychological change. You're not thinking on that level when you're walking the streets crying or looking up at the ceiling for hours. Your body will feel how it feels, especially when you're alone. During that period, I didn't have what psychedelics people call 'containers' to contextualise my altered states in my everyday life: places, relationships, face-to-face conversations, community, movement, or rituals.

Donald Winnicott coined the phrase 'the holding environment' in reference to the physical holding that a baby needs from its caregivers' arms, as well as the highly attuned attention that provides a figurative container of care.[9] Within this holding environment, the baby's mind is shaped by its relationship to its environment and everyone around it.

Infantilising ourselves and our needs can be limiting, but we do continue to need holding environments throughout our lives to give us context. For those of us who lived alone during Covid, we lost our holding environment; we were not held. Meanwhile, those of us who lived in couples or families lost the broader holding environment of community in which those units must always stay nested. If we define mind not as the subjective experience that's happening inside your head, but an intersubjective process that happens between us, as Dan Siegel does, you could say that we literally lose our minds when we lose our relationships. No wonder so many people lost their minds during Covid.

My psychotherapy during the lockdowns of 2020/21 was a holding environment, and it was valuable and meaningful, but it was one hour a week, and that was not enough. Though I'm a proponent of psychotherapy, and my therapist friends are some of the wisest and most skilled people I know, I'm uncomfortable with the pedestal that this largely inaccessible model has been put on by the middle classes. And given our mental health crisis, I don't think any sacred cows should be beyond scrutiny.

It's worth reflecting on what exactly it is about therapy that does seem to help. Multiple studies have suggested that more than any therapeutic modality, it's the quality of the therapeutic relationship that determines successful outcomes.[10] In keeping with this, I like R. D. Laing's definition of psychotherapy as the attempt of two people 'to recover the wholeness of being human through the relationship between them.'[11] This speaks to the power of therapy at its best; to the almost mystical role that a good therapist can play in healing. But given how many people are in crisis and in desperate need for holistic, foundational help with their lives, not just their psychology, I don't think expensive, one-on-one therapy is a sensible model at scale. There are many ways to recover the wholeness of being human through relationship; many structures the psych industry will never be incentivised to promote because they don't involve psych professionals. Things like team sport, communal music and dance, group retreats, youth clubs, excursions into nature, the fostering of a pedagogic culture of collective learning and value sharing. Again, I think my squeamishness about how twee this all sounds speaks to my sense of loss and longing for such a culture.

I felt that longing profoundly during the pandemic. Despite making strides in my MDMA work with Rachel and Jonathan, without broader relational containers I continued to struggle. Religious scholar Huston Smith expressed scepticism of psychedelics' innate ability to transform mental health without the structures to hold them:

> Human history suggests that without a social vessel to hold the wine of revelation, it tends to dribble away. In most cases, even the most extraordinary experiences provide lasting benefits . . . only if they become the basis of ongoing work. That's the next research question, it seems to me: What conditions of community and practice best help people to hold on to what comes to them in those moments of revelation, converting it into abiding light in their own lives?[12]

Most of us, in lockdown or not, do not have the kinds of social vessels that our ancestors could rely on (in places of worship and community), and without them, healing is a slog. As much as we may want to let go of our old strategies, our systems are unlikely to relax unless we're able to demonstrate that we are supported. Somehow, we have to convince the worried parts of us (parts who are stubborn for good reasons), that it's safe not to worry any more.

Personifications of this dynamic repeatedly popped into my imagination, both on and off psychedelics, as I wrote in December 2021:

I was reflecting on how much better my OCD was and I suddenly felt disconnected from myself. I had a mental image of myself as a kid, when my OCD started, and I had an upswell of grief at the thought of leaving that girl alone in the past, as if to recover from OCD would be to somehow abandon her. As if my OCD had somehow been keeping her alive. The thought of leaving her there devastated me. There's a part of me that can't let go because I have to keep her alive. How do I leave OCD as a survival mechanism behind, and bring her with me? I don't know.

It wasn't just her. There were ghosts all over the place. In another recurrent imaginal vignette, I would go back as an adult to my childhood home and find my child-self standing in my bedroom. I would encourage her to leave with me, but even though things in that house were incredibly tough, she'd insist on staying.

I found myself in a double bind that I didn't know how to break: a child-self desperate to let go of her strategies, blocked by the adult who didn't want to abandon her; an adult-self desperate to move on, blocked by the child who was fixed to the spot. All these gaps across which reason couldn't reach.

How can you talk your psyche out of a situation when its motivations are opaque and the glimpses it gives you are internally contradictory? Clearly, something remained beyond me, some mysterious resistance to healing whose logic I couldn't fathom. Something above my head or at my roots? I didn't know what or where, but I knew that I wasn't done looking.

Roots

It's 2022. I've come to meet Betty. I'm happy to see that the stone grave is well kept and that there's a conifer growing next to it. Nearby, the Black Mountains form the high dark wall between England and Wales. Two of my old schoolfriends have driven me here and are waiting a little way off. It's a cold, grey day.

One day in late 1946, George and Catherine Cartwright, who had been trying for a baby since they returned from New York, walked into an orphanage in Birmingham and asked the nuns which of the infants most needed a home. They took a sickly baby, my dad, into loving arms, and his birth mother Betty, having come in every day to breastfeed him since she was forced to give him up, never saw him again.

The page of the story turns on two letters that sit side by side in our family file, both written to the priest who ran the orphanage. One from grandma Betty in May 1946: 'I am only eighteen, Father, and my parents won't allow me to take him home.' And one from grandma Catherine Cartwright eight months later: 'He has made us very happy,

Father, he is a very loveable child and seems to be quite happy and content.'

I like to think this longed-for motherhood sent restorative love back into Catherine's own childhood, to the moment she tried to wake her mother, with whom she shared a bed, from sleep. As a woman, Catherine would still remember the question she'd asked over and over that morning. 'Why are you so cold, Mam? Why are you so cold?'

By the time Dad learned of Betty's existence, she'd been dead twenty years, having died of breast cancer, aged 60. She'd gone on to marry, had had four more children and had moved here to the Welsh borders, hopefully a breath of fresh air from the factories of Birmingham.

I want to hear 100 voices roaring with the love and loss of these forgotten exchanges. I want to be frightened by their faces etched on masks looming out of darkness, so I can feel what they felt. I want to dance in firelight for three nights straight until blood streams from my nose and I can't stand up and it's done. But how, when we've lost the collective rituals and practices that celebrate the extended self of

our ancestry? How, when I'm a godless individual, siloed in time, do I say *thank you* to my grandparents for the love that lit up my parents' baby brains like lanterns? How do I let myself be guided by them? How do I be resilient like them? How do I embody their stories and make myths with them? I want to work steel like Grandad George, bring ideas together like chains. I want to be an escapist like Papy André who outfoxed the gatekeepers. I want to be a rock like Betty. But how?

I don't know. But I can stand by this stone grave, at the edge of the stony Black Mountains, on this cold, grey day, with my friends waiting a little way off, and close my eyes and think of the roots of the conifer down there. Where Betty used to be. Not separate from the rocky ground, the ground not separate from the soles of my shoes, from the structure of the bones in my feet, knees and head. Not separate from my heart where my ancestors' stories beat. Not separate from my mind which can build those beats into the pillars which hold up the roof of this book and give my story structure.

Back story

'The process of initiation can be likened to a sacred catastrophe. A holy failure that actually extinguishes our alienation: our loneliness; and reveals our true nature: our love. That is why we seek initiation, to heal old wounds by re-entering them, in order to transform suffering into compassion.'[1]

Roshi Joan Halifax, Buddhist teacher

I was about 7 years old when I first realised that we were broke. I remember the exact moment.

At lunchtime at school, we all had to queue up in the dining hall, filing past a dinner lady at a trestle table whose job it was to collect £1.20 off each kid, except from the free-school-meals kids, who were exempt. I remember the smell of the smiley potato faces, overcooked cauliflower and chocolate custard. The shiny grey floor tiles covered in scuff marks from gym shoes.

The kids filed past the dinner lady one by one and gave

her their coins as they usually did. She said 'thank you' to each of them in a sing-song voice and ticked their names off a list. When it was my turn, I stood in front of the table not knowing what to say, or what to do with my arms, conscious that the classmate on either side of me was witnessing the conspicuous absence of a transaction. The dinner lady ticked my name off the list and filled the silence with a smile. I'd done this countless times, but on this particular day, that smile unsettled me. I realised it was a different smile to the one the other kids got, like she knew something about my life that I didn't. It was the start of a drawn-out process of emotional echolocation, during which I created an internal picture of what it meant to be broke and what society thought about that.

It took me so long to realise because a lot of my parents' friends from church were poorer than we were. I saw inside houses that were more cramped, damp, and chaotic than ours, and met people whose predicaments were far worse. When Mom was well, she sometimes worked as a carer for the housebound, and, as paying for a childminder was out of the question, I would go along with her on her jobs, chatting to her clients while she did the housework. No matter the mess or the stink or the grumbling that greeted her, she never averted her eyes, never lost her patience, never lost the lilt in her voice. At the end of each shift, I got to leave those places holding her hand, and I think, even as a tiny kid, I knew that meant I was inestimably wealthy, which is why the dinner lady's sympathy – yeah, that was the word – was so confusing.

Exposure to social adversities dramatically increases the

likelihood of a person becoming seriously distressed and getting diagnosed with a mental disorder. This has not only been a consistent finding of research for decades, it's one of the most trustworthy and universal intuitions we have: when bad things happen, we feel bad. The conclusions of the UK Poverty 2022 study shouldn't surprise us. Adults in food-insecure households have higher risks of developing mental health issues, and debt can place huge stress on a family's mental wellbeing.[2] Financial insecurity can lead to serious distress, and serious distress can lead to financial insecurity, each factor amplifying the other, leading to further distress and further insecurity and a knot that is immensely difficult to untie. I've seen many friends and family go through versions of this cycle:

Broke.
Unable to find a job, leads to depression.
On the dole.
Get a job.
Still broke.
Meaningless work leads to more depression.
Too depressed to work.
On incapacity benefit.
Broke.

According to research conducted by the Samaritans, 'As area-level deprivation increases, so does suicidal behaviour. Suicide rates are two to three times higher in the most deprived neighbourhoods compared to the most affluent.'[3] 'Men in the lowest social class, living in the most deprived areas, are up to ten times more at risk of suicide than those in the highest social class, living in the most affluent areas.'[4] An NHS study found that children (aged 5–16) with a mental disorder were more than twice as likely to live in a household that'd fallen behind with payments and that in 2020, children living with a psychologically distressed parent were nearly three times more likely to have a mental disorder themselves[5]. Other factors – including poor education, racial discrimination, disability, poor diet, urban development and displacement – can negatively affect mental health and poverty in complex ways, each issue compounding the others. All of these also compound with an individual's biology, creating a snowball effect in which single root causes become impossible to identify. Ethnic minorities in the UK are more likely to live in low-income households (the poverty rate of Bangladeshi people in the UK is more than double that of white people).[6] People with long-term physical health conditions and disabilities are more likely to have mental health problems: one study found that 54 per cent of people with learning disabilities have a mental health problem.[7] Transgender and gender non-conforming populations are also far more likely to experience both poverty and mental health problems.[8]

The causal relationships at play here, and how they are felt within the hearts of individuals and communities, can't easily be measured; nor, I don't think, is measurement a prerequisite for understanding. We know and deeply trust through our experience that human beings are responsive to the conditions of the environment in which they live.

I was recently walking with a close schoolfriend called

Sally in a beautiful abandoned gravel pit, now covered with trees, at the edge of the Black Country. Her dad had been given a diagnosis of schizophrenia in the 1990s, and had been in and out of Bushey Fields, the same psychiatric hospital as my mom, at around the same time. He was given electric shock therapy, which she said changed him forever. When we were little girls, we didn't understand what was happening to our parents, but we knew it was something awful, the thing we heard whispers about in the playground: the 'nervous breakdown'. It was a phrase that gave me the creeps. Linguistically, both words are what's known as spondaic, i.e. having two stressed syllables: *nerv-ous break-down,* which is why it sounds like being clubbed four times over the head.

Though speaking about mental health in terms of nerves is now back in another guise through the popularisation of the polyvagal theory, and through practices that soothe the nervous system (like yoga, tai chi, and breathwork), usage of the phrase 'nervous breakdown' dropped off sharply after the 2010s.[9] It was seen as old fashioned and less scientific than the new brain sciences. But in its wooliness, 'nervous breakdown' was arguably a more helpful framing than the pseudo-specificity of diagnosis, in that it didn't tag anyone with a reductive explanation of their problem, and it pointed to mental health problems as all-body problems. It also carried with it an implication of reactivity – people usually had nervous breakdowns because life had got too much, not because they had an indiscriminate illness in their brains.

As an article in *The Atlantic* put it, 'For 80 years or so, proclaiming that you were having a nervous breakdown was a legitimized way of declaring a sort of temporary emotional bankruptcy in the face of modern life's stresses.'[10] We assumed that the person who'd had a breakdown must have been facing some immense difficulties in their lives. I think generally we do still assume that of someone who's been hospitalised with mental health problems – that at some point, they experienced something terrible. It's compassionate and common sense to wonder, as the trauma adage goes, what happened to them, not what's wrong with them; but in twisted psychiatric logic, we've been led to think that it's stigmatising to wonder this, since it fails to view mental illness in the value-neutral way we view many other illnesses.

Here's anthropologist Roy Richard Grinker, author of *Nobody's Normal: How Culture Created the Stigma of Mental Illness*:

In most studies – this turn to see psychiatric conditions as brain disorders has actually exacerbated stigma. There is less stigma when we see [poor mental health] as a complex result of many forces, when we see it as a response to environment, when society takes some of the blame, or something else . . . like a war, or a virus, a pandemic. There's more stigma when we see it as: 'this is a problem within that individual'.[11]

I've thought a lot about what might fill the gap if medicalised language rescinds. We already have some words – emotional crisis, spiritual emergency – and even simple words like alienation, disconnection, heartbreak and grief capture much about the nature of what we're led to believe is an epidemic of brain disorders.

Over the years, Sally and I have spent hours talking about the predicaments of our respective families and our shared histories. She likes to remind me of the time I set her school books on fire. I like to remind her of the time she hid cat shit in her dad's slippers. No fucking wonder our parents had *multiple nervous breakdowns*. Our laughter petered out as we walked the top bank of the gravel pit, looking over the canopy of trees below, and we were quiet again.

'What makes you think that mental health problems are responses to hardship?' I asked her.

She paused and thought about it. 'Just from knowing people,' she said.

I thought it was a brilliant answer. One which spoke to a deep implicit knowledge about mental health that we've been taught to mistrust. Through its promotion of a disease model of emotional suffering, our mental health system has reduced, as well as over-complicated, something that, in the process of writing this book, I've discovered that I always believed: emotional suffering is, at root, understandable. Even if a person's thoughts and behaviours seem irrational, disproportionate, extreme, even harmful, they make sense at some level.

Science (true, sceptical, holistic science) is an essential tool in understanding what makes us suffer and flourish, but in speaking to several scientists while researching this book, I've often encountered dismissiveness towards this kind of implicit knowledge. Many scientists seem to trust what people report under study conditions more than they trust what people say around pub tables or what they whisper on pillows.

Part of my healing has been getting my head around how,

as I was assessed by dozens of psych professionals of various stripes over fifteen years, my mental health was repeatedly taken in isolation from the broader social conditions that were the soil of my childhood. After the initial 'history taking' part of a psychotherapeutic relationship, these things were almost never discussed, let alone integrated. In *Pure* I actually extolled the virtues of this wilful ignoring of context. I said how much I liked CBT because it was interested in hows and not whys. 'Whys' are painful, so it was understandable that I didn't want to go near them. But I have learned the hard way that 'whys' will always come back around to bite you.

~

'Though many people would say we've adopted a more biopsychosocial approach, psychiatry is still dominated by biological thinking,' psychiatrist Dr Gareth Knott told me. 'It's not just driven by psychiatrists, it's also driven by patients. A lot of patients want diagnoses and medication. If anything, I'm often telling patients that changes to their work and social lives would be more effective than medication.'[12]

Dr Knott is part of the South London and Maudsley NHS Trust, which offers the widest range of mental health services in the country. He works in a community in Lambeth, a financially deprived area of the city where, before the pandemic, about 43 per cent of all children lived in poverty.[13] He painted a picture of a busy clinic where patients typically have very serious mental problems and precarious hand-to-mouth lives, and like many of the thoughtful psychiatrists

I've met, he's troubled by the medicalised legacy of his profession. 'If someone's homeless and they're drinking too much because they're cold at night, what is an antidepressant going to do to help? It's really, really bad out there.'

I told Dr Knott about my work with psychedelics and meditation and how these had helped me find meaning.

'The whole meaning-making thing can sometimes come from a privileged place,' he said. 'Some people are not able to engage on that level. They're just trying to get through life without worrying about self-actualisation . . . Look at psychotherapy. Long-term therapy is primarily private. It's expensive. It's a middle class phenomenon. People from low income and minority ethnic backgrounds, who suffer more and need the most help, often can't access or afford it.'[14]

Given the right social and psychological support, I think even people with very serious mental health problems are able to find meaning, if not through altered states, then through community creative expression, art and music. But Dr Knott is right – it's a privilege to have that support. The healing quest of a middle-class white woman is not a roadmap that the most disadvantaged people in society can easily follow. Nor is it the help they immediately and desperately need. When you're trying to keep the wolf from the door, there's no room for quests. No space in the head for anything but bills. No margins in life for leisure.

'Unemployment grinds you down,' my dad told me recently when I asked him about his redundancy in 1990, when I was 4 years old. Dad had started working when he was a boy, as a farmhand on a pig farm. Later, he became a lab technician, and progressed to become a cameraman and eventually a documentary director at the Central studios in Birmingham. A job that he said gave him purpose, intellectual stimulation and a sense of accomplishment at being able to provide. When Thatcher privatised the networks, he was put out of work along with six hundred colleagues. His redundancy cost him the financial comfort he'd established for his family, and plunged him into the maddening bureaucracy of the benefits system; back into manual labour (a car factory, this time) and the working-class life he'd been born into. He applied for sixty jobs in the first six months and received sixty rejections.

'The situation was grim. Your mom decided to seek work as a care assistant as we were living from hand to mouth. As I ground through my daily job searches, I started to drink vodka in the mornings. People at Mass were giving me money,' he said. 'My overwhelming mental state was one of frustration. I had to face down PTSD whenever something sparked in me the reality of what I had now become. I once saw [a former colleague] at Euston station when going for an interview and had to control my emotions. It was the man who had given me my redundancy cheque.'

I went to the Job Centre with Dad many times as a kid and saw on people's faces, grey as the carpets, what unemployment does to a community. Dad recalled one occasion at the dole office that particularly upset him: when he witnessed an illiterate man in his sixties, who'd had a rough life doing manual work in factories, being asked by an officious and condescending clerk why he wasn't reading the daily papers to find work. 'How degrading,' Dad said. 'He was being treated like detritus, not a human being.'

'What helped you cope?' I asked.

'The strength of our marriage. Prayer. And having previously had to cope with the trauma of my cancer.'[15] (He'd nearly died of Hodgkin's disease as a newlywed in 1976. My eldest brother and sister were babies at the time.)

These things live inside you forever. They don't get processed in therapy like things get processed in factories, as psychologist James Hillman said. I wouldn't ever want to *refine* them. Their coarseness was instructive. There is, to borrow language from Buddhist teacher Roshi Joan Halifax, a sacredness in the catastrophe[16] that has shaped me.

I've always been drawn, for example, to writing that blends bitter with sweet. I can pinpoint the childhood experiences which I suspect created that sensibility. Like the time I visited Mom in Bushey Fields at Christmas and saw the festive cards that the patients had made and stuck to the notice board. I was destroyed and uplifted at the same time. In a way, healing has been a hunt for these between-tones and aesthetic thresholds, the places where wholeness emerges in the same beat as heartbreak.

It's worth looking at the privileged place from which my meaning-making has come, and how this has factored in my wellbeing. I have the privilege of being financially well off, white and straight. I have my own flat in which I can do as much therapy as I like. I've been lucky enough to land a job that gives me not only a sense of purpose and creative satisfaction, but the resources to invest in any modality I want to try. Retreats. Psychedelic guides. Conferences. Bio-trackers and gadgets. All this has cost tens of thousands. I couldn't have pursued my healing the way I have if I'd still been broke. Then there are the other things that go along with this privilege, like access, contacts, and confidence.

There's something problematic about WEIRD people telling the story of their healing as though it were an accessible path to everybody. A narrative that says 'if I can do it, you can do it too' is often cheerfully blind to the social advantage that has helped along the way. As far as I can tell, almost everyone on the trauma-healing landscape – gurus, psychonauts, yogis, influencers – are middle class, and I see few of them citing this as a factor in their healing. If we don't see the impact of our good fortune, we may chalk all of our wellbeing up to the efficacy of the modalities with which we've been working.

A breathwork routine in a spacious, light-filled apartment that you pay someone to clean, is not the same in a space that is dim and cold. Gratitude practice, done however diligently, won't pay the bills. Not everyone can get time off work for therapy. It is reported that 1.9 million households in Britain can't afford access to the internet,[17] so no YouTube yoga videos or guided meditations for them.

The market has pulled off an impressive magic trick that we might not have noticed, since it has done so over a span of a few thousand years: it turned the basic fundamentals of human wellbeing into luxuries with a price tag. A living space with lots of sunlight and nearby greenery comes at an eye-watering premium. Healthy food has been rebranded as a superfood for the elites. Human touch of various kinds can be bought for an hourly rate. Adventure days and daredevil experiences rouse our adrenaline, give us perspective and make us feel alive. Our distant ancestors had these things on tap, for free, constantly rubbing shoulders with each other, surviving, facing down danger and taking up space, with the sounds of nature omnipresent. Now, we pipe those sounds out of plastic boxes as we try to sleep. Self-care has become a convenient meme for capitalism, not only because it almost always involves buying something – from bath salts to gym shoes to smoothie-makers to haircuts – but because if we're all doing self-care then we're doing the community's job for it.

'A lot of politics is about delegation. Politicians are delegating responsibility on to doctors and social workers,' Dr Peter Kinderman told me. Dr Kinderman is a professor of clinical psychology at the University of Liverpool. He takes the view that the disease model serves the government well, because it scapegoats social problems that call for policy changes on to individuals. Funding and promoting psychiatry, he thinks, enables the government to give the impression that it's doing something to help people.

And, as he put it, 'we go: "No, that's not what we meant. Actually, we meant can we have universal basic income, please? And can we have double the minimum wage and can we have a four-day week? Can we have synchronisation of the school day with the working day of parents? And can we have universal childcare? And can we have proper accountability for crimes against women?"'

'Treating mental health problems as social problems would mean a radical overhaul of the status quo,' I said to Dr Kinderman. 'It would mean actually dealing with things like unemployment and abuse and discrimination. Do you think that the disease model has been so popular because it's just easier to say to a person, "This problem exists inside your head"?'

'Yes. The social changes that we would need, both as a community and as individuals to protect and promote our mental health would be big steps. And that worries me, because if you say that the "epidemic" of antidepressant prescriptions, especially in socially-deprived areas, should be addressed as a social problem . . . I'm not sure that that's going to happen in my lifetime.'[18]

~

There was something I couldn't get my head around. Something which, during my clamber out of the mental illness paradigm and my search for an alternative, didn't add up. I was adopting two schools of thought at once. On the one hand, I was adopting a trauma-informed world view, which says that how you think is a result of negative experience. On the other hand, I had been deepening my meditation practice, going on yearly retreats and adopting a Buddhist world view, which says that negative experience is a result of how you think. One hand: attachment wounds, traumatic memory, authentic self. Other hand: non-attachment, memory as construct, illusory self. 'That bad thing shouldn't have happened to you' vs 'nothing is objectively bad'.

What was confusing and interesting was that I was equally enamoured of each way of looking. It was helpful to think of some experiences as objectively bad and of people's reactivity being a natural follow-on. But I couldn't square that with the equally appealing idea that we all have agency to change ourselves and that our reactivity is the source of our suffering.

After several years of psychedelics and meditation practice, I found an awareness starting to creep in around how reactive I was. When my emotions were raging, I was able to notice: this reaction is not commensurate with the situation. *I feel fucking awful, but this situation is not objectively bad.* Having one step of removal in this way started to give me a sliver of control over my reactions, and that control fed back into my perception of the experience.

It was there in stoicism. 'If you are distressed by anything external, the pain is not due to the thing itself,' Marcus Aurelius wrote, 'but to your estimate of it; and this you have the power to revoke at any moment.'[19] Later, it was there in Shakespeare, as Hamlet, imprisoned by his thoughts, declares: 'for there is nothing either good or bad but thinking makes it so.' His next, lesser quoted line, 'O, God! I could be bounded in a nutshell, and count myself a king of infinite space; were it not that I have bad dreams'[20] is a haunting reminder that it's our psychology, not objective constraint, that imprisons us. Yet isn't it also true that some people live in circumstances that we could all agree are miserable; circumstances that do, and really ought to, affect how they feel? If you're bounded in a nutshell, isn't it natural and right that you would feel, well, bounded in a nutshell?

CBT is widely considered a 'gold standard' treatment for anxiety and depression.[21] It, too, usually points to the conclusion that what needs changing most in a person's life is how they think about life. CBT can be helpful, and at its best it is nuanced and relational. In my opinion, it can also be dogmatic. If handled by a therapist who doesn't understand trauma, the relentless message – rationalise your irrational beliefs, undistort your cognitive distortions – can dismiss the underlying cause of these phenomena and place the task of change squarely at the individual's door. Again, I wonder if one of the reasons that CBT has been so enthusiastically promoted by the government is because the wham-bam, standardised fashion in which it's often delivered tacitly upholds the philosophical position that people in adversity ought to – and have the power to – change their feelings about adversity.

After several years of CBT, I came away with a fairly narrow and unskilful modus operandi: manage your responses to your thoughts, be resilient. All well and good. Only, sometimes situations didn't call for my resilience – they called for self-soothing, or getting the hell out of there. If 'nothing is either good or bad but thinking makes it so', then thoughts like 'this feels off' were not an intuitive warning sign to act, they were to be dismissed as faulty thinking. I was often so focussed on changing my unhealthy internal patterns, it was hard for me to identify unhealthy external situations and relationships.

This 'personalisation', Dr Kinderman said, is another legacy of the disease model. 'Resilience is useful. But, for example, I don't think that women should develop resilience against men attacking them in the street, I think men should stop attacking women in the street . . . There's resilience, there's also identifying the nature of the problem in society and addressing the problem, rather than just focusing on the individual.'[22]

As professor of sociology Dr James Davies put it, '"Resilience" is a sneaky neoliberal trope. It frames, as a psychological virtue, painful endurance of circumstances from which others benefit at your expense . . . being "resilient" can be crucial. What I am critiquing here is the ideological use of the term in schools, workplaces, oppressive settings, e.g. making a virtue of tolerating circumstances better defied.'[23]

I ran my quandary past Dr Kinderman. Have my mental health problems been the result of my circumstances or the result of the way that I think about my circumstances? He introduced me to the idea of 'the social determinants of perception', meaning that perception itself is partially determined by environment. On reflection this sounds obvious, but it hadn't been to me. I was so used to thinking in binary terms about the mind inside my head and the world outside it; of my thinking as a product of the machinery of my brain, quite separate from the environment.

'It's a powerful psychological finding that we do have agency,' Dr Kinderman said. 'But the way we discharge our agency is shaped by how we were brought up, how we've been treated and the things that have happened to us.'[24] In other words, the extent to which we're able to have dominion over our behaviour is also partly determined by the stressors we've been exposed to.

These ideas were freeing on a couple of counts. One, it was intellectually satisfying to see an apparent dichotomy with which I'd struggled, blend and soften on closer inspection. Two, it introduced a more skilful flexibility into my self-therapy that stopped me clinging too tightly to any one way of seeing my story. A sort of 'yes, also' approach. Yes, bad things happened that led to my suffering. Also, I have an active role in the perpetuation of that suffering. This means I get to keep all of the compassion and causal common sense of the trauma model, and keep all of the agency of the stoic one. Viewing myself as a victim of negative circumstances helped me move towards my pain, while viewing myself as the source of negative patterns helped me not get stuck there. Eventually I found I could lightly hold both views at once, since both were true. And since, for the traumatised person, pain has the contradictory quality of wanting to be known and to hide at once, it's apt to have a double-ended tool in the toolbox.

'The trauma model can be extremely helpful,' said Dr Knott, 'but it has its problems as well. At some point, probably, a person needs to let go of trauma. While understandable and adaptive, a victim narrative can be limiting.'[25]

'I totally agree,' I replied, 'although I would say that the current tools on offer, like CBT and SSRIs, are not very good for treating trauma. You can't choose to let it go if it's there.' In my experience, trauma can only be let go once its stuck potential is expressed and harmony begins to restore. Until the process of reacquaintance with *what wholeness feels like* begins, it is exceptionally hard to exercise power over your emotions.

Perhaps it's not only a case of deciding what model to use for which person, but what model when. It's not that CBT isn't useful, it just wasn't appropriate for me at the time it was prescribed. Nor is a rake appropriate when an industrial digger is what's needed. Once I started to have experiences of mastery, safety, and agency through psyche-delics, that's when talk therapy and practices like meditation started to unlock for me, when my nervous system was finally calm enough to allow rationalisations and reassurances to be heard.

~

Bushey Fields serves some of the most deprived areas in the Midlands, areas which, not coincidentally, have the highest rates of mental ill health. Once, when I was visiting Mom, a patient repeatedly asked me for the time, then verified it with the watch he was wearing. It was funny the first few times – we both thought so – but then it didn't stop, and became awkward, and I didn't know how to handle it. It was a confusing place. The strip lights were always on. Time didn't seem to exist there.

I remember that Mom would talk about how she felt patronised by the psychiatric process, and about how self-righteous her psychiatrist was. When she told him that talk therapy was not helping her feel better, he scoffed at her and suggested maybe the problem was her attitude. I didn't realise that what Mom was describing was the very problematic finger-trap dynamic in psychiatry – the more you struggle, the deeper in you get; the more you oppose, the more this is evidence of your pathology. Opposition in this dynamic can never be justified, grounded, and rational, it is always oppositional, defiant, and pathological. Trauma narratives can also serve the same purpose. 'It's too easy for therapists,' says Allen Frances, 'to assume that anytime the patient is upset with the treatment, or upset with the therapist, it has to do with a re-enactment of the past . . . rather than it being perfectly appropriate anger or upset due to the fact that the therapist has said or done something that's been hurtful.'[26]

I just wanted Mom to stop being stubborn and do what the doctors said, because they were the ones with the qualifications and they knew best. The medicalised story of suffering is insidious – it gets into people's lives and relationships, influencing the way we frame the ones we love. The rational bit of me knows that I was a kid and that it wasn't my job to understand these things; the emotional bit of me feels that I let her down. I would come to know this doctor–patient power dynamic well in my own interactions with doctors, where the authority was almost always on the other side of the table. (I've been scoffed at myself more than once.) A psychiatric relationship that affords the patient no control and treats them as anything less than a collaborative partner runs the risk of recreating the conditions of powerlessness that brought the patient through the doors in the first place.

Dr Kinderman says that control, or lack of it, is central to emotional distress: 'The social conditions in which we live and the events that happen, constrain the parameters of control that we have. If you're poor and you're lonely, you have fewer ways of controlling the variables that are important to your wellbeing.'[27] This hits on a very important distinction: it is lack of control, rather than lack of money, that is at the heart of adversity.

Robert Waldinger, one of the lead researchers in the Harvard Development Study, the longest running study into human flourishing, has found that once a person's basic material needs are met, happiness doesn't increase with wealth. The happiest study participants are all people with high-quality personal relationships 'who invest in things beyond themselves and who really care about having things live in the world . . . that are not about *I*, *me* and *mine*, or even just *my family*.'[28]

Most of us will know happy people who have very little wealth, or wealthy people who are miserable. I met a lot of the former when I was growing up. I meet a lot of the latter in the entertainment industry. Though the struggles of wealthy people may not be as immediately sympathetic, it is a wretched kind of suffering to realise that money can't heal your wounds.

~

My mother never identified with her diagnosis of bipolar disorder, though that didn't seem to matter to those charged with her care. I wonder what avenues that diagnosis opened up and justified in the treatment decision tree? Many times, over many years, she was sedated, hospitalised, and prescribed cocktails of powerful antidepressants, antipsychotics, and anticonvulsants. The meds were not short-term crisis interventions, they are life-long.

Meanwhile our family received none of the support that would have tackled the problem from the ground up and made her life easier; support that every family deserves: help looking after children, an education system that meets children's needs, fairly-paid work in the community, freedom from worry about the utilities being cut off, breathing space from stress, access to physical space that facilitates our most powerful conduit to resilience – community. Mom needed circles of people, circles of generations, surrounding her every day, keeping her in orbit. We had none of that.

A social worker would come to the house sometimes when Mom was back home. It's extraordinary to think that an hour a week of structured conversation, plus a psychiatric review every few months and a dosage increase, was considered a satisfactory offering. That someone whose mental health doesn't improve under such conditions can get categorised as 'treatment resistant', placing the onus on us for our resistance, rather than on the treatment for its inadequacy.

As I watched all of this as a sensitive little girl, and listened through the walls when the emergency doctors came, I didn't understand what I was seeing and hearing. There was a layer of horror that I wouldn't grasp until well into my thirties: the horror of a government that effectively uses psychiatry to launder social problems through the minds of individuals, delegating its weightiest responsibilities to the most vulnerable people.

As Dr Davies put it:

What should be a national or even international conversation about where neoliberal policy has corrosive emotional effects in our public sector, in our schools, in our workplaces, in our universities, and in our wider economy, instead becomes a conversation about the growing epidemic of mental illness in all of these domains of modern life, a conversation often draped in sanctimonious and conspicuously pious calls for more mental health provision, less mental health stigma, more mental health conversations – ever louder calls for more of the failing same.[29]

As we've seen, trauma-informed and psychedelic healing models also run the risk of performing a kind of delegation of their own, reducing vast social context to attachment wounds, holding a magnifying glass over single issues, single relationships, single nodes in a system, and neglecting the wider systemic whole in which those nodes are nested.

Derek Summerfield wrote that suffering is objectified and turned into

a technical problem – 'traumatisation' – to which technical solutions are seen to be applicable . . . This view of trauma as an individual-centred event is in line with the tradition in both western biomedicine and psychology, which is to regard the singular human being as the basic unit of study.[30]

I did experience abandonment as a kid, but I don't think it was as simple as separation anxiety from my mother, though that was indeed immense. It was also the abandonment of a family by a state and the abandonment of a region by a country. Our sense of separation from those we love is indivisible from a set of broader separations: separation of our species from nature, separation of our spiritual selves from meaning and purpose, and of all of us from the strangers who surround us.

Medical anthropologist Adam Aronovich, who has worked extensively with ayahuasca in indigenous contexts, explains how droves of Westerners come to the Amazon on their healing quests, oblivious to the fact that, for many locals, the whole idea of an individual healing journey is a strange concept.

> If a person is feeling sad or anxious, it is very unlikely that the community will tell that person there's something wrong with your brain. Rather: how are your relationships? Are you feeling held by your community? Are you engaged in life in a way that feels meaningful for you? Is there anything that we can do to make you feel more integrated? . . . For all the technology that we have and the pharmaceutical advancement that we have, when it comes to mental wellness or psychic wellbeing, Westernised cultures usually fare much worse than traditional societies . . . It says a lot just not only about the failure of hegemonic, mainstream, biological psychiatric approaches, but also the importance of tightly knit communities.[31]

For several years, as I thought I was making progress on my 'healing journey' through a radical shift in thinking, I didn't realise that I had merely replaced the medical model with a similarly totalising trauma model; replaced old language with new – 'OCD' with 'trauma', SSRIs with psychedelics. Yet I was continuing to treat my problems like they ended at the edges of my body in a solitary pursuit of happiness. My healing journey was, like our entire wellness culture, selfish, egocentric, and inward looking.

'What if you were to take all that machinery of integration that you're using to integrate yourself and you turned it on the world?' says cognitive scientist John Vervaeke. 'What if you took all of that capacity to glue things together and you exapted it on the world? That's when the world comes alive to us.'[32] This 'radical decentering'[33], as he calls it, is a crucial and undersold aspect of getting better from mental health problems. Do we have to deeply understand ourselves before we can engage in bigger social issues, or does an engagement in social issues deepen our understanding of ourselves?

It was only when I came to understand my family's pain as reactive to what had happened to us, that I counterintuitively started to feel better; started to hope that there could soon be an end to the constant volatility of two steps forward, one step back. Our popular healing culture can encourage us to reduce our family members to pawns in our psychotherapeutic narratives, and to create fixed ideas about who they are and how that has shaped us. To some extent this may be helpful. But it can also cause us to overlook our loved ones' complexity and depth. I had been worried about writing this book for fear of exposing my family to my pain, but by bringing them into the process, the shared pain was transformed into a force for connection.

As I sat in front of my dad reading his handwritten notes about redundancy and the decline of the Midlands in the 1990s, ('shops closing, clapped-out trains, shortages of hospital staff'), I learned new things about his life and cried without hiding my emotion from him. 'I'm so sorry that you had to go through this,' I said. It's not a coincidence that this most healing moment involved putting my own naval-gazing aside and stepping into someone else's heart. As Zen Buddhist Henry Shukman said, 'there's something about deep wounding that can be a pathway to deep love. It's a beautiful thing when the wound becomes the doorway.'[34]

Ultimately, it was an immense relief to take some of the energy that I had for so long directed towards interrogating internal psychological mechanics and turn it towards interrogating external social mechanics. It was only when I started to realise that healing is not personal, but political, that I paradoxically found a new intimate understanding of myself. If we can bear to look, the healing codes we need are right there in the stories closest to us.

~

By early 2022, I had a clear intuition that I wanted to do mushrooms again. Nothing had ever taken me as deep or dark and I sensed that there was treasure in that darkness. But I was terrified. The idea of experiencing something as harrowing as watching Mom disappear into the cosmos again? I didn't know if I could do it.

But I was better informed and better connected this time and I figured I could rebuild my relationship with mushrooms in a gentler way. Over two years I had been getting to know two mushroom guides, Val and Beth, whom I trusted. With their support I decided that I would do a 'hippie flip' – a mix of MDMA and psilocybin. I'd heard that the MDMA can lessen the likelihood of a bad trip, softening some of the hard edges, keeping you more grounded in your identity, and making you less likely to be shot into oblivion.

Almost immediately after taking the drugs, my motor

function was blasted. I couldn't raise my head, and my limbs had no coordination. (I hadn't felt like this since I snorted ketamine at a house party thinking it was coke, and had been found on the bathroom floor, flailing like an upturned beetle.) MDMA mixed with mushrooms: this was some fucking magic! I realised the reason I couldn't move was because I was a newborn baby, and with that realisation I was *gone*, deep into an all-body, all-mind reconstruction of infancy. It was an incoherent world of struggle and discovery, with no references, no words, no map. Just roiling textures, sounds and sensations. Soon, I opened my eyes and my vision filled with light as I had the first thought that I ever had: 'Mommy.'

My self-consciousness had burst over a threshold and I was now in relationship with everything around me. I spent the next five hours growing through toddlerhood, learning to crawl, then sit. At one point, I asked Val to help me put my socks on (because I was two years old and didn't know how). At the peak of the experience, while still a child, I was as big as the universe, batting planets around like tennis balls. It was, at least at that point, the most exquisite and astonishing thing that had ever happened to me.

In the aftermath, as with past trips, I felt significantly worse before I started to improve. Psychedelics can often do this: inflame inner conflict rather than soothe it. The inflammation was ultimately helpful, in that it showed me where my defences were and why. But feeling better was not an inevitability. I was left wondering whether this time I'd finally flown too close to the sun and done irrecoverable damage to my psyche. Day to day, the sensation in my chest was increasingly intense, as though I was physically being dragged in different directions. 'I feel a moving towards and a pulling away at the same time. I want comfort but I fear it,' I wrote in my journal in April 2022, perhaps giving voice to the preverbal infant I met while hippie flipping. 'To let love in would be to realise how much I needed Mom, and that feels dangerous. When you have trauma, love and pain hold each other at arms' length. How do I bring them together? You can't feel one without the other.'

Clearly, I was still holding something back.

Val hosted group mushroom retreats and had told me their door was always open, but I'd been too scared to say yes. I didn't want to let go of control in a group. What if I went crazy in front of them? What if I humiliated myself? What if I pissed myself? What if someone else's trip terrified me? What if someone vomited? What if I vomited? What if they told their friends what a freak I am? What if I blurted out something that I later regret? What if I hurt someone? What if they hurt me? What if they judged me?

My questions pointed to the exact nature of my personal oblivion: letting my body be vulnerable in a group of people. My years of very public memoir writing had been a shadow play of the vulnerability I was still avoiding in real life; the confrontation I couldn't continue to avoid if I ever wanted to arrive at resolution. I had made myself into a walking fortress to keep people out. It was people, after all, who had taken Mom away. People who had taken Dad's job away.

My fears, as they often do, showed me the North Star I had to follow. If I ever wanted to find my way out of my maddening nonlinear maze, I would need to prioritise and commit to the single most powerful healing resource we have, and the only one that really counts. Not some old wisdom repackaged as self-help, not some new-fangled psychotherapeutic modality. Not psychedelics, but community.

I am because I party

'When you separate mind from the structure in which it is immanent, such as human relationship, the human society, or the ecosystem, you thereby embark, I believe, on a fundamental error, which in the end will surely hurt you.'[1]

Gregory Bateson, anthropologist

The minibus stopped.

'We're here,' someone said.

I couldn't see where because rainwater was streaming down the window. I stepped off the bus onto a flooded mud path that led to a single-storey ochre building.

I was in Côte D'Ivoire in West Africa, visiting a school for animist priestesses, where girls from the Akan culture are initiated into a sacred order of wisewomen. Through elaborate ceremonies, they dance themselves into altered states of consciousness, during which they say they are possessed by spirits whose energy they dramatise and express, and whose will they interpret. This sacred sorority dates back many centuries, with roots in the old Ashanti kingdom, which spanned parts of Côte D'Ivoire and modern-day Ghana.

I had been wanting to learn more about a traditional community practice that cultivates non-drug-induced altered states. My own first mystical experience had been sober, and I'd had other non-drug-induced trips since. On one occasion, on a retreat, I'd started having spectacular auditory hallucinations of birdsong when my head hit the pillow at night. An entire woodland in song, different calling patterns and species, constantly generating, never looping. It seemed that, below my conscious awareness, my system had made a note of these sounds as I'd been meditating during the day, and was then able to play them back to me in perfect mimicry. Many traditional societies know this and live this: we don't need psychedelics to have extraordinary internal experiences, we just need the right practices to facilitate their unfolding.

I had been reading about the ways that the practices of different traditional societies may hold clues as to how mental health problems can be prevented. Since falling into psychedelic and alternative healing culture, I'd been bombarded with talk of rituals, ceremony, and holding space. I wanted to see how space was held by people for whom ritual is an integral part of life.

Accessing the sacred ceremonies of another culture is complicated and sensitive. You need to be vouched for, trusted by and introduced by someone local, especially if you're a white Westerner visiting a country that's been historically oppressed by white colonialists, and where systems of oppression still continue today. I was lucky to be introduced to a friend of a friend who, having built relationships with locals through several trips exploring voodoo in West Africa, was gathering a small group for a trip to Côte D'Ivoire to learn about the trance, divination, and mask traditions of the Dan and Akan people. Each elaborate ceremony would last many hours, encompassing music, dance, singing and masks, and involved the whole community, from elders to babies. Sometimes, during harvest or ancestor festivals, or when someone dies, these ceremonies last days.

The fact that we were present would inevitably alter the context of what we saw. Visitors can't experience these rituals in their full authenticity, and so it should be. The symbols, costumes, rhythms, and movements have long aural histories, spoken in local languages, that are idiosyncratic and rooted to each specific place and people, and much is lost in translation. According to our guide, a member of the Dan ethnic group, sacred knowledge can't be performed, it can only be experienced by the initiated.

In the villages I saw ways of life that I didn't see in London: people living in direct contact with nature; many generations socialising together; children being cared for communally, with groups of mothers, sisters, aunts, and grandmothers all sharing caregiver duties; groups of children playing and fighting without parental supervision in public spaces, with young children looking after toddlers. (There's a tendency in psychedelic and trauma healing circles to generalise and idealise traditional societies, but life is difficult on many fronts in Côte D'Ivoire. Nearly half the people live below the poverty line, sanitation and water quality is poor, and discrimination against women and gay people is common.)

We entered the sitting room of the school, dripping rain-water everywhere. The head of the order, addressed as Mother, was waiting. She explained in French that typically the girls who arrive there (some are sent by families to which they will return, some are orphaned, some abandoned) have what the West calls mental health problems. Our guide, as he translated for the English speakers, did the seemingly inter-national sign for psychological disturbance by waving his hands around his head chaotically.

I asked about this later that day. Where would these girls go if they didn't come here? Are there mental health hospitals they can visit? Psychiatrists? With a shake of the head, the guide explained that the framing of my question doesn't make sense in Ivoirian culture: 'Hospitals and doctors are for when you have a broken leg or you need a vaccination against a disease. If someone here gets disturbed, it's seen as a spiritual problem with spiritual solutions. Psychiatric disease is the disease of the Westerner.' (According to the World Health Organization's World Mental Health Atlas[2] of 2017, in that year in Côte D'Ivoire there were 0.13 psychiatrists per 100,000 people, roughly 30 for the entire population of 23 million at the time.)

Girls arrive at the priestess school between the ages of 9 and 12, and their spiritual education lasts three years. When they graduate and become initiated into the order, they can take up official roles in their villages or set up private practice, where locals will seek their advice for health complaints and spiritual problems. While still at the school, they live, work and play there, in community. Purity is a central concept. The girls must purify their spirits and void themselves of defilements so that they become a clean receptacle through which to channel spirits.

As a liberal atheist, this idea of voiding yourself through spiritual purification makes me uneasy, and yet, though the framing is different, I'm struck by how similar it sounds to notions with which I'm familiar: the idea in Buddhism of transcending ego in order to experience emptiness. The idea in psychedelic culture of returning to wholeness by ridding yourself of trauma.

In this part of Africa, animistic religions blend with Christian anthropomorphism. The priestesses believe in spirits that inhabit rivers, forests, and mountains, as well as in a series of archetypal characters. At the end of a small, dark room, stood fifty or so wooden statues, each representing a different spirit. A hunter, a mother, a warrior. While the notion of surrendering to the will of external spirits may sound passive, there seemed to be an emphasis on the girls' special agency in their work. An unmissable message was written in French in large letters across the courtyard wall: '*Tu n'es pas le maître de mon destin.*' ('You are not the master of my destiny.')

A single cowbell sounded from somewhere in the commune. It was time for the ceremony. Hushed by a nervous energy and not knowing what to expect, our group took our seats on plastic chairs arranged around a central dance area. Everything was quiet, save for the rain, and this piercing bell, played by Mother, who seemed to be summoning the others. Over the next fifteen minutes of constant ringing, the people in the commune prepared for the ceremony – put down their chores, slid on their shoes, retied headdresses – until twenty-five or so people had assembled on the chairs at one end of the shelter, mainly women, from babies to elders, and a few men.

One by one, people playing maracas and wooden blocks joined in with Mother's bell. The women sang while three men began beating huge drums with sticks. I felt my jaw fall open at how astonishingly loud the drums were. A baby sat on a woman's knee, seemingly unfazed by the volume. I tried to guess the beats per minute – as fast as psytrance certainly. After forty or so minutes, I started to feel lulled by this incomprehensible wall of sound and my thoughts grew quieter. Some aesthetic experiences are so huge, layered and insistent, they make your self sit back.

Summoned by the blowing of whistles, three priestesses aged in their twenties and thirties, walked in procession into the dance area. They wore red beaded hats and colourful fringed skirts. They draped themselves in shells and tied strings of bells around their waists and ankles; their skin was covered in clay.

Rounds of dramatic synchronised dancing began, with each round representing possession by a different spirit. The priestesses waved bunches of human hair, spun in circles, put on white sheets. At one point, a little girl with a sash tied around her waist, a trainee priestess, received a lesson in how to dance like her elders, following them in a circle, mimicking their swaying. While the atmosphere was sacred, it was also casual. Occasionally a couple of women would share a chat or joke and laughter would ripple. A kid at the back was bored and looking at his phone. The priestesses broke out of dance sometimes to hug the instrumentalists. As people's levels of engagement rose and fell, there seemed to be an organically maintained core of activity over several hours. It was no one person's responsibility to keep the ember of the ceremony glowing, its emergent energy was distinct from any one individual.

I hadn't thought that the drumming had anywhere to escalate to, but as this story reached its climax, the drummers increased the pace and volume. With sweat dripping from their faces, the three priestesses spun in ever-faster circles and threw back their heads, causing the fronds of their skirts to splay hypnotically. The percussive shells and jingling bells on their waists meant that my sound and vision became a single sense. The lead dancer rubbed charcoal on her face and produced an enormous knife. She started to stagger and tremble, her eyes crossed as she seemed to enter an altered state of consciousness. She spun around screaming as she held the knife against her belly, enacting a confrontation with a death spirit, as a wave of exhilarating fright moved through the room and little kids took in the scene with wide eyes, housed in the laps of adults where it was safe to feel afraid.

The waves started to roll back, the drumming slackened, the last round of music and dance petered out as the priestesses staggered to a standstill and the story came full circle, with the sound of the single cowbell which slowed, then stopped.

Afterwards, I thought about that little trainee priestess with the sash tied around her waist. I don't know what adversities had brought her through the doors, or what kind of life would await her upon graduation. But in her education, she was seemingly being told a very different story about what distress means than a Western child is typically told. One tradition evokes spirits as causal agents. The other, mental illnesses. Putting aside for a moment the content of these respective stories and looking at the practices they facilitate, I don't think the latter necessarily represents progress. While it may give sceptics pause, the proposition made by these animist priestesses facilitates a series of beneficial procedures: communal living, participatory dance, singing, coming-of-age rites, and connection to a higher purpose. These are the babies in the bathwater that the West threw out with religion, the fundamental unmet needs at the core of our mental health crisis.

The Sacred Design Lab at Harvard Divinity School identifies three things we all need for fulfilment: belonging (the experience of being deeply known and loved), becoming (developing the gifts we can give to the world), and beyond (experiencing ourselves as part of something bigger). It posits, 'The more we go hungry for meaning, connection and purpose, the more we act from isolation and despair. This plays out in the way we live, love, work, and lead. The problem is soul-deep. So, too, must be our response.'[3]

What response does our medicalised mental health story facilitate? In the UK, we'll take a sensitive, socially isolated kid who's under constant online scrutiny and exam stress, whose parents are too overworked to be emotionally present, and rather than tell her that the problem is in the world we've built, we'll tell her that the problem is in her brain or her thinking. This leads her, not to the noisy, expressive, embodied community practices that might help her feel her soul-deep connection to the world, but to static encounters at doctors' desks and corrective individual therapy and medication. While these kinds of interventions may sometimes help in the short term, clearly they are not helping to improve the mental health crisis generally. According to UK charity Young Minds, in 2018–19 nearly a quarter of 17-year-olds reported having self-harmed in the previous year.[4]

I came back from Côte D'Ivoire feeling moved by the glimpse I'd had of various ritualised modes of expressing emotion through embodied storytelling. It served as a reminder that there is not just one psychology but many ethnopsychologies; that 'mental illness' is not universal, but part of an ontological claim about what it means to be a human being, and that people with different ways of life make different claims. I wondered if a more pluralistic approach to mental health might be a balm for the system of incentives and siloisation and lack of professional humility that makes the UK mental health system so slow to change.

Theories that fit the Western psycho-psychiatric model of the world have, over time, got so bedded-in that they've started to feel like reality. It's been challenging for me to admit that theories that have been personally useful and that I would've once considered globally applicable, like attachment theory, are not necessarily helpful for everyone, or even for most of the world. Child psychology expert Nandita Chaudhary, who's conducted case studies on child rearing internationally, points out that in cultures where children have many multigenerational attachment bonds, the primary caregiver model of attachment theory bears little relevance.[5] Far from a monolithic reality, the latter could be seen as symptomatic of the burden that atomised family life puts on mothers and fathers, who are often isolated from extended family and peer support.

Disruptive states of consciousness might be able to help us step back and conduct an auditing process of our cherished ideas, since they show us the way we model the world, and that these models are not the same as reality.

~

In spring 2022, my mental health was still oscillating. I'd seen glimmers of what connectivity could feel like, but I would often still find myself crushed by numbness or lost in mind fog. My body would still tense up when it was touched. I was still waking up with heart palpitations a couple of times a week. All hallmarks of trauma.

I had decided to prioritise community above everything, in hopes of soon feeling safe enough to do a group mushroom retreat, and I was looking for ways to engage my body in things like dance and breathwork. But because we've decimated the wisdom and the physical spaces out of which communal traditions might have evolved organically, 'intentional' alternative healing practices can feel clunky and derivative. As inappropriate as it is to globally export Western healing models as though they were universally applicable, it is also problematic to generalise the context-specific practices of traditional societies and co-opt them into an individualistic healing culture. Things like 'mindful movement', 'voice empowerment' classes and trauma release workshops, often have a certain tonal signature, a well-intentioned but uncomfortable hodgepodge of South American and Eastern influences, led almost exclusively by earnest middle-class white people who have the time and luxury to pursue these kinds of careers.

The UK does, however, have a blueprint for a genuinely organic mass healing movement in our recent past: the rave culture of the 1980s and '90s. In 1993, combined attendance at jungle, drum & bass, house, and techno parties in Great Britain was 50 million.[6] It was a primarily working-class, racially diverse movement that attracted seekers from all walks of life. It had big electronic beats and altered states of consciousness; people who were there often describe it as having been a spiritual, transcendent cultural moment. In the post-industrial West Midlands where I grew-up, ugly, angular between-zones – carparks, disused warehouses – became gathering places where people could unite and let go. Places where 'the weak become heroes', as Birmingham artist Mike Skinner said.[7] It was in this tradition, on dancefloors, surrounded by people and movement, where I felt at home and ultimately did most of my integration.

One night in spring 2022, at an Ibizan club called DC-10 I found myself nodding blissfully on MDMA for five hours to punishing techno, holding the hand of my oldest friend. I couldn't tell where the sensation in my hand stopped and that of my friend's began. I couldn't tell where the music ended and the ache in my chest began. Sound and sensation were the same in a single field of consciousness as the bassline blended with my heartbeat and seemed to pulse from there. Inside became outside and vice versa.

Most weeks I danced sober, at day parties, or at my local ecstatic dance community space. Sometimes so intensely I entered altered states of consciousness. After a couple of hours, dripping with sweat, when I was unable to tell which of the many hands waving in my vision were my own, when I didn't know if the thuds I was hearing were from my feet or someone else's, I would feel my sense of self start to expand, as though we were dancing not as individuals but as a collective body. This effect is what psychiatrist Dan Siegel calls differentiation and linkage[8]: feeling both like a defined autonomous body and a broader social body at once, a somatic integration, which mysteriously facilitates psychological integration and the ability to approach old problems in new ways.

'If the self were defined as *the interiorisation of community*,' wrote James Hillman, 'then the boundaries between me and another would be much less sure. I would be with myself when I'm walking with others. I would not be with myself when I'm walking alone. And "others" would not only include other people. Community, as I see it, is something more ecological, or at least animistic. A psychic field. And if I'm not in a psychic field with others – with people, buildings, animals, trees – I *am* not. So it wouldn't be, "I am because I think" (*cogito ergo sum*, as Descartes said). It would be "I am because I party" (*convivo ergo sum*).'[9]

Anthropologist and systems theorist Gregory Bateson offered us a related idea when he said that our minds are not a closed mental system but an 'eco-mental system'.[10] In *Steps to an Ecology of Mind*, Bateson posited that Darwinism left something crucial out of the picture. The unit of survival, Bateson said, is not individual + species, it is individual + species + environment[11], meaning that the world is not something external, it is part of our psychology. Those of us growing weary of the hyper-individualism, divisiveness, and tribalism of today's consumerist healing culture are offered a fresh vision in these more inclusive redefinitions of self and community.

On a seven-day group silent meditation retreat in 2022, I realised how tapped in I'd become to a broader feeling of interconnectedness. Midway through the retreat, I took a very small dose of mushroom chocolate then took a walk in some woodland. I saw something that, until that moment, would have seemed impossible: the shape of every individual leaf on every tree, all at once. The edges of leaves which I would've thought too thin to pick out, the movement of one leaf as distinct from its neighbour. I saw more hues of green and blue in the sunlight than I knew existed. Ivy tumbling in exquisite high definition from the upper branches. Fern tendrils emerging in fountains from the understorey. Everything swayed and was softly spectacular in this leafy wonderland. Charismatic, exciting, and inviting. My sense of clarity was astonishing. Like me, the wood was alive. Every bit of it was changing all the time, just like the community of organisms that is my body. I realised this was what a wood actually looks like when the reducing valve of my own mental model loosens; when I'm no longer holding up the predictive map of reality that shields me from reality itself. Emergent from this experience was the sense that my mind was no longer locked in my head but branching out in every direction into the woodland, where it could be effortlessly carried. I was no longer called upon to hold up its weight on my own.

This is what I mean when I say 'show don't tell'. Don't get bogged down in psychological theories and self-help or the pros and cons of different types of therapy. Look for life's entactogens, the things that put you in touch with others and the ecosystem; prioritise finding the experiences that show you through your senses the inalienable fact of your own belonging. You can't just be told that you belong or that you matter or that you are a part of things. You have to be shown. The belonging will feel new, but also familiar, and that's how you'll know that it's always been there.

It was through these experiences of deep connection of various kinds, that I slowly started to trust myself and others enough to do a massive psilocybin journey, surrounded by people.

~

The group sits in a circle and we set our intentions. Some intend to heal, others to surrender. There are tears and respectful silences and nods of understanding.

I take 5g of mushrooms in chocolate, and when it hits, it hits brutally hard. I suddenly find myself rolling and twisting through a harrowing vortex of gut-coloured tubes. I am just about holding on to a single sentence that ropes down from the surface:

This is profoundly terrifying.
This is profoundly terrifying.
This is profoundly terrifying.

I feel like I might throw up. Facilitator Val helps me walk to the bathroom, where I sit, bent double over my knees, sobbing, disorientated, shattered.

'Don't close the door, don't leave me,' I beg Val. She leaves the door ajar and waits outside, checking in occasionally to make sure I don't hit my head on the sink. I try to stand. 'Have I done something wrong?' I say to Val, clinging to her.

'No sweetheart, you haven't done anything wrong,' she says, holding me. 'You're doing an amazing job.' She leads me back over to my mat and tucks me in.

From here I am taken back into darkness. Colossal columns rise from the centre of the earth. Among them, a green phosphorescent orb appears. It speaks in a synthetic woman's voice as it floats away from me: 'We now find ourselves at the beginning of human consciousness. You're about to discover the depth of human happiness that is possible beyond thought.'

There is no 'me' witnessing any of this. No way I can agree or disagree to follow her as she floats into the darkness. This all just happens, depersonalised from any biographical context, in a void.

Next thing I know, I am me again. Back in my body, lying on the mattress with my blindfold off, aware of my surroundings, the flowers in the centre of the room, the massive mandala on the wall, every surface smudging and sparkling, so pretty.

I think I've pushed through the darkness to the other side when something catches my eye. Another member of the group, a woman in her fifties, is lying a few feet away. Horror washes through me as I see her as a corpse. The skin on her face is sunken, the eye sockets hollow and enormous, the teeth protruding horribly from the rictus mouth. I want to look away but I don't. 'Show me what I need to see,' I say to the mushrooms as I stare down at this corpse's face, sweating with fear. Then the realisation hits me like a sonic boom. 'I thought Mom was dying. When I saw her in those states. That's why I was so afraid,' I say. With that realisation, I feel the fear drain away and move into the past. The corpse face disappears and I'm once again looking at the serene face of a friend.

I start to feel a warm glow in my chest slowly build, and do not fight it. I lie my head back and feel a lovely stretch down my throat and collar bones, before my heart, slowly, blissfully, wrenches wide open, pouring light out into the room as three decades of love that I've shut out pours in. I understand it all at once: all of the relationships of my life. The grudges I've held. The tallies I've kept of the ways I've been wronged. The way I've starved friendships of oxygen. The sniping and the judgement. The way I've closed my heart the instant I've felt anger or fear or loss. I understand it all. The faces of people I love appear and disappear. I love you. I am sorry. I forgive you. None of that bullshit matters. *I am all in. I want you to know that I'm all in.*

Then, another shift, as I suddenly grow younger, into a little girl, and in the single most blissful moment of my life, I am flooded with a realisation, which I speak in a child's voice: 'Mommy's okay.' I hold my head as I weep. 'Mommy's okay, she's okay. Mommy's okay'. I say it again and again and again.

A benevolent, grown-up presence is embracing me and assuring me that this is true. 'She's okay, baby girl, she's okay.'

I rock myself. I press my palm against my forehead and laugh as a little girl. 'I didn't know. I didn't know. But she's okay. Mommy's okay now. She's okay.'

In the fourth hour, reality comes back together like oil droplets on the surface of water. I remember where I am and how old I am. I look around the room at the others, who are still deep down in their trips, and weep with love for them. That's when the effervescent laughter starts.

'What a bunch of assholes.'

INT. BARRY'S BEDROOM, LONDON - DAY

Barry is lying on his bed looking at the ceiling.
Yesterday he did a psychedelic trip and today he's
depleted. A precocious 12-year-old boy enters, wearing
Bermuda shorts and a tie-dye T-shirt.

                    BOY
          Hey, Barry.

Barry doesn't look at him but grunts.

                    BOY
          I know you hate me but I need to
          talk to you.

                    BARRY
          Go away.

Barry rolls over and faces away.

                    BOY
          You know the more you shut me out
          the worse this is going to be?

The boy sits on the edge of the bed. This irritates
Barry.

                    BOY
          Do you remember the time when you
          were 9 years old and Mom was really
          sick and she locked herself in the
          bathroom and there were no other
          grown ups around and you didn't know
          what to do?

On Barry as he remembers.

                    BOY
          Do you remember the next week at
          school, when all the kids had to
          write down what they were sorry for
          on little bits of paper? Then the
          priest burned the papers so that
          God would forgive you?

                    BARRY
          I remember.

                    BOY
          Do you remember what you wrote?

Barry exhales.

                    BARRY
        'I'm sorry for making Mom cry.'

The boy, strangely mature for his age, nods. He
lets this land.

                    BOY
        I was paying very close attention
        to you around that time because I
        knew you were struggling. I knew
        that you were strong and that you'd
        bounce back if things improved.
        But they didn't did they?

                    BARRY
        No.

                    BOY
        They got worse didn't they?

                    BARRY
        Yeah.

Barry pulls his knees up to his chest, he looks
small and childlike.

                    BOY
        Do you remember the day in France
        when you were looking out across
        the ocean with the weird feeling
        in your chest?

                    BARRY
        Mm.

                    BOY
        That's when I stepped in.

                    BARRY
        Stepped in?

                    BOY
        I'd already tried some strategies
        with the skiving and the faking
        illness. But I knew then it was
        time to bring out the big guns.

Barry might already know the answer but he asks
anyway, in a small voice:

                    BARRY
        What big guns?

                    BOY
          Do you know who I am?

Barry is silent.

                    BOY
          Please look at me.

Barry won't look.

                    BOY
          This won't end if you can't look.

Barry turns to look straight at the boy. The boy
stares back.

                    BARRY
          You're my OCD.

A beat as something is unlocked. The entire scene
pivots and shudders as roles are swapped. Barry sits
up and seems bigger while the kid seems smaller. The
boy bursts into tears, suddenly childlike.

                    BOY
          I just wanted to protect you.
          I'm so sorry I ruined your life.

Barry looks at his own hands, feels his face and
realises something. A rush of protectiveness sweeps
through Barry. He crouches to cuddle the boy.

                    BARRY
          I'm a grown up, you don't have to
          protect me any more.

                    BOY
          I wanted you to think about someth-
          ing else. I didn't know what else
          to do.

                    BARRY
          You were so clever.

He kisses the boy's head.

                    BARRY
          I'm sorry I wasn't there to help
          you but I'm here now.

                    BOY
          It's all my fault.

                    BARRY
          Look at me.

The boy won't look.

                    BARRY
          Please look at me.

The boy looks. Barry stares back.

                    BARRY
          It wasn't your fault, okay? You
          don't have to be sorry.

The boy's lip quivers as he nods his head.

                    BARRY
          You can stop those strategies now.

                    BOY
          You've told me that a million
          times. How do I believe you'll be
          kay if I stop?

Barry has an idea. He breaks the embrace, stands and
reaches out his hand.

                    BARRY
          You don't have to believe. C'mon.

The boy takes his hand hesitantly.

                    BOY
          Where are we going?

                    BARRY
          I'm going to show you your life.

Their voices fade out as they leave the room, holding
hands.

                    BOY
          Okay.

                    BARRY
          I think you're gonna like it.

Kill your darlings

'All tales, then, are at some level a journey into the woods to find the missing part of us, to retrieve it and make ourselves whole. Storytelling is as simple – and complex – as that. That's the pattern. That's how we tell stories.'[1]

John Yorke, Script editor

Writers will tell you that a book is never finished, only abandoned, and I think the same must be true of trauma healing. Any end point would be an arbitrary mark on a continuum, and there's always the possibility of stepping backwards. But there has been a meaningful and dramatic difference between the frightened mess I was when I went to that meditation retreat in 2017, and my present day-to-day.

Writing in 2023, I have been out of regular psychotherapy for two years, having spent the preceding seventeen years having weekly or fortnightly sessions. Seventeen years when my life was almost unbearable, with thousands of intrusive thoughts a day. They've now reduced by around 95 per cent. I haven't had a suicidal thought or urge to cut myself in years. The content of my dreams has softened and I sleep better. Nightmares are rarer. Having used it as a social crutch for years, I've almost completely lost my taste for alcohol. Slowly, the good days became more numerous, the bad days far less. Eventually, the good days became so numerous and the bad days so manageable, they were no longer noteworthy. My diary entries petered out in 2021, then stopped. Every week I enjoy feelings of spontaneity and authenticity, and experience joy upon noticing some novel sense of connectedness with the world, and intense gratitude and disbelief about how much my inner life has changed. I often find myself blindsided by banalities: people are good, I'm lucky to be here, the evening light is beautiful. The most noticeable shift has been my newfound ability to be uplifted by the presence, eye contact, voices, and touch of others. My nervous system feels alive.

When I look back on the way I described 'feeling better' after my intensive CBT ten years ago, I notice a tone of resignation; a kind of radical acceptance that frightening intrusive thoughts would always be a part of my life; a steely resilience in the face of the biological hand I'd been dealt. I didn't realise that I was regurgitating a stock script that had been handed to me by psych professionals who themselves seemed resigned, having seen so many intractable cases. The script said that OCD is a chronic condition and that in all likelihood, I'd be managing symptoms for the rest of my life. My bar of expectation was low. I thought the best I could hope for was mastery of my psychological responses to anxiety, an anxiety that would always return because that's what my brain was like. It would've seemed fanciful to hope that one day the anxiety would be so soft and infrequent, it simply wouldn't call for a response.

While it does seem true that childhood trauma can be released, never to return, we remain responsive to stress throughout our lives. During the writers' strikes of 2023, I felt a tangible drop in my resilience. I was isolated from my team and lost my means of earning money, at the same time that rising interest rates skyrocketed my mortgage. I'd once watched Dad lose the career he'd loved because of massive industrial forces like this, a career that'd once seemed secure. Healing doesn't mean we become impervious to broad social stressors; if anything it shines a compassionate light on our vulnerabilities to them.

During that time, I also got a bad bout of Covid and was alone and immobilised for two weeks. My obsessions, compulsions, and nightmares returned, quieter than the old times but there. If another person were emotionally unruffled by a fortnight of solitude, would we explain the difference between me and this hypothetical person as mental illness? What would we be measuring in such a comparison? Can environmental conditions be measured at all or are they inescapably relational? It's not just the environment that matters, but what the environment means to each individual. An empty house might mean different things to different people, perhaps depending on the meaning that it carried in the past. Contemplating having a mental illness can be easier than contemplating how hard it is, in an individualistic society, for even the most privileged among us to get our need for community support met. Something will try to fill the gulf if we can't.

There was a cornerstone moment when I realised how much better things were. I was lying around and laughing with a guy I was dating. It was late and we had to be up early but I didn't care how tired I'd be the next day. I wasn't worried about how I'd look in the daylight. I had no confusing or horrifying intrusive thoughts and no tearing sensations in my chest. I wasn't living any life but this one. I felt energised and safe. When we kissed, no part of me kicked out of orbit. All of me was able to stay fully relaxed for the first time in someone else's arms. The time window had closed. I was no longer feeling everything through its changeless frame.

The progress had been gradual, but the step-change happened after my group psilocybin experience – what some people call a 'breakthrough journey'. Until then, I hadn't realised how scared I had been of fully letting go in front of a group of people. In the end it was this surrender, this utmost vulnerability and utmost trust, as much as the drugs themselves, that healed me. It was the risk of abandoning myself into the care of others, and seeing that this care could be counted on, which enabled my system to explore parts of my psyche I'm not sure I could ever have reached on psychedelics alone. As though I first needed to trust that there was a village of people on the surface holding the other end of the rope before I could be confident enough to explore the depths.

A few weeks after that journey, I'd had a follow-up conversation with facilitator Val, who had helped me off the bathroom floor when my sense of self was in pieces and I was shaking and sobbing, unsure if I'd ever come back together.

'What do you want to talk about today?' Val had said.

It's a question I'd been asked hundreds of times by therapists and I'd always had a list of things on the agenda, to maximise my therapy minutes and squeeze the last bit of self-actualising value out of the healing project.

'Do you know what?' I said. 'I don't think I want to talk.'

Val mirrored my smile.

'That moment of realisation that I had: "Mommy's okay, Mommy's okay, Mommy's okay." I was scared that I would lose it and that it would drain away like so many other insights I've had. But so far it's stayed. It's the first time in my life I've ever had that "nothing else matters" feeling. You know that feeling? Like everything is fine as long as I have this?'

Val nodded.

'It didn't cure me,' I said. 'But it left me feeling that I can handle all of that bullshit, because I'm a grown-up and it's not that deep. Somehow, magically, none of that matters too much now that I have this knowledge that she's okay. Happiness isn't the right word for how I feel. It's tenderness. It's like an ocean of tenderness.'

We were both crying by then.

'So I don't feel like I need to talk any more, I need to go out and live my life. I've done enough. There's nothing more to talk about because she's okay.'

And for the first time in hundreds of hours across seventeen years of therapy, I left a session after only a few minutes. I wasn't a project any more, there was nothing pressing to do.

Meditation teacher and psychotherapist Loch Kelly offers a simple instruction for guided meditation practice, a question to ask ourselves when we're lost in thought: 'What's here now, when there's no problem to solve?'[2] I wasn't going to find out 'what's here' by talking about it. I needed to go out and experience it. And in a way, this is where things started not ended.

~

Did you ever do that thing when you were a kid, when you counted the seconds between the flash of lightning and the thunderclap? The longer the gap, the further away in miles the storm was. When a bright flash was followed instantly by a big boom, you knew the storm was right over your head. It's a fun little calculation to give to kids. While mindfully paying attention to the counting and to the sensory experience of light and sound, the mind is less likely to race with thoughts about how scary the bangs are.

I wonder whether people write books about their struggles to serve a similar function, to take their minds off the storm until it passes. Or maybe at an unconscious level our systems understand that the stories we tell about ourselves have the ability to feed back into the lives we lead. That it could be the integrative action of storytelling itself, as much as any therapeutic intervention, that heals. In an essay called 'Life as Narrative', American psychologist Jerome Bruner wrote:

> I believe that the ways of telling and the ways of conceptualizing . . . become so habitual that they finally become recipes for structuring experience itself, for laying down

routes into memory, for not only guiding the life narrative up to the present but directing it into the future. I have argued that a life as led is inseparable from a life as told.[3]

In other words, if you don't have a recipe, you can write one. If you don't know where you're going, it may help to imagine and reimagine what your map might look like, until imaginary roads home become real ones.

Imagination is difficult though. If you've never had prolonged periods of feeling well, secure, and connected, then trying to imagine how that feels is like trying to imagine a new colour. You'll often hear people who've recovered from mental health crises say they could never have imagined achieving xyz positive thing or feeling xyz positive way. We should take this seriously. Often, being well can be literally unimaginable. If challenging things have happened to you over many years, things that disrupted your ability to trust that everything's okay, your system will struggle to find a blueprint feeling in the past to build a positive vision of the future. Altered states have led me to believe that we all have within us a blueprint feeling of love and belonging to fall back on, even if the way we live so often obstructs our access to it. And that we all bear the responsibility of carrying that blueprint for others when they can't trust that it's there.

For years, my relationships – which is to say, my sense of self – were inseparable from an overwhelming fear of loss, and in the latter stages of getting better (I use the past tense gingerly), I clung to that fear because I thought that if I stopped being afraid I'd lose my relationships, and therefore my self. Western psychiatry, with its deficit model of healing as a reduction in symptoms, a negation of a bad thing rather than an emergence of a good thing, failed, in its lack of imagination, to help me resolve this double bind. My strategies were destroying me. And yet I couldn't give them up for fear of being destroyed.

In this book I've explored different definitions of healing. Healing as engagement with community. Healing as an integration of ancestral stories. Healing as a newfound ability to feel bodily sensations. Healing as a thawing of frozenness. Healing as a non-resistance to pain. Healing as a swapping of unhealthy disruptors for healthy ones. Healing as a reacquaintance with the inner child. Healing as political not personal. Healing as a decentring of self. Healing as a newly awakened receptivity to love. Healing as breaking into the boardroom and discovering that the heart committee are not malevolent saboteurs but the most tender and creative parts of you, whose counterintuitive workings now make perfect sense, who have strategised for you and hauled for you. Who always had absolute faith that you'd one day stride in, take a seat at the table and run this bitch.

The medical model had taught me everything about being ill, and almost nothing about *being*. Being a healthy, well-adjusted grown-up, who has a sense of agency and accomplishment, whose relationships are infused with a sense of security that reaches right down to bones, heart, lungs, and tummy. It's something you really have to feel to know. So I made a list, in case I ever forget, of what being well feels like.

- Trusting that you are held as a loved person in the hearts of others
- Feeling like you're worth protecting
- 'Right here' and 'right now' feel okay – you don't need to escape
- You can rest in your body
- You want to be in your body and not anywhere else
- The sensations inside your body are familiar, they feel like 'you'
- Feeling like you belong at home
- Your breath comes and goes easily in your belly
- Feeling that you are a cherished part of a group
- You can receive praise and believe it
- You can receive criticism and use it to build better relationships
- Feeling like you have the power to impact other people's lives positively
- Your anger burns clean
- Feeling soothed by the touch, words, and gaze of others
- Understanding what everyone always meant when they talked about 'life'
- Your emotions are safely contained in your body – they have a bottom and a top
- Feeling like your opinions are valued and sought out by others
- The tone of your inner voice is compassionate, especially when you make mistakes
- Trusting that you are worthy of kindness
- You have a strong sense of the boundary where your body ends and the world begins

- You feel in control of that boundary
- You trust that sleep will bring you rest
- If you let go, you won't spin away

The one thing that all meaningful definitions of healing have in common is connection, and another way of thinking about connection is closing the gap between things. Gaps have come up a lot for me: the gap between my rationality and my feelings; the gap between the grown-up woman I was supposed to be and the frightened child I felt; the gap between what research says about the causes of mental suffering and what the public has been led to understand. Healing for me has meant trying to bridge some of these gaps and the awful dissonance that thrived in them. Though there's an exception to this pattern, since in a very concrete sense, healing could be conceptualised as the *opening* of a gap.

~

In 2017, with no trauma knowledge, and no insights into the responsive function that my symptoms were performing, I went on a meditation retreat in California in the hope of curing my OCD. I found myself blindsided by a non-ordinary state of consciousness during which the symptoms of my lifelong illness temporarily subsided. At the time, my inner life was clouded by a storm of anxiety and obsessive thoughts, which raged constantly. My teacher on that retreat, Joseph Goldstein, gave me a very simple instruction for whenever I noticed I was lost in thought: 'Begin again.' It has been helpful for when I've been lost in stories, too.

I've sat three retreats since, collectively spending more than a month in silence – not much compared to experienced meditators, but enough to be persuaded of the singular value of the meditation cushion as a lab in which to observe how the mind–body system works. Over the years, I started to put my finger on the 'bottom up' pattern that I'd once tried and failed to explain to my CBT therapist. I could see it clearly: my thoughts were not triggering anxiety as I'd been told; my anxiety was triggering thoughts. It was hard to spot, because the separation between the flash of physical anxiety and the boom of the associated story was a constant and terrible light and sound show, raging right above my head. The sensation ('anxiety') and the meaning ('something bad is happening') were identical. I could never have imagined teasing apart the association.

Two of these retreats were taught in the tradition of a brilliant Buddhist teacher called Rob Burbea. Rob's talks helped me through my rocky 'two steps forward, one step back' phase, and his voice became a constant when everything else was oscillating. In a lecture called 'Heart Work' he stopped me in my tracks when he articulated something delicate and important that I hadn't found words for.

'You can actually catch an emotion being built,' he said. 'There's a sensation in the body and a thought gets connected to the sensation. [It] gets interpreted in a certain way, and bada-bing, there I have it. *I'm in. I know this one.*'

Below the radar of conscious awareness, he was saying, body sensations that would be otherwise neutral can be overlaid with a thunderous story, and the more that that association gets laid down, the more it's likely to be made in future – a connection through habit.

'We don't block any of this as we watch it,' Rob continued. 'We don't try to stop any of it. We are just allowing everything in consciousness. And in that very allowing, the thing doesn't get constructed.'[4]

The thing doesn't get constructed. I love this twist. It turns on its head the psychological framing of trying to overcome the negative emotions that stand between us and wholeness. Here, Rob is saying that you can simply observe the prior state of unfettered wholeness from which emotions emerge, picking up on the theme with which I've become enamoured while writing this book: that healing is a restoration of something that was always there, rather than a destination at the end of a journey. That sometimes the hardest job is to rest back and observe that wholeness in ourselves. Our love and connection to each other can be unbearable and excruciating in light of the way we live, but it's there to be felt if we dare.

In 2022, I was fascinated when I heard an interview with neuroscientist Lisa Feldman Barrett in which she discussed the constructed nature of emotion. The brain, she said, doesn't know the causes of your feelings, 'it draws on past experience to make a guess at the cause, it's doing it predictively. So when your brain guesses that the cause of a tug in your chest is anxiety (because in the past, in this context, in this situation, that's what it was) then your brain is constructing anxiety. That's how you experienced that tug in your chest. But you can deconstruct the feeling of anxiety into just a mere tug in your chest. That's what mindfulness meditation teaches you to do.'[5]

So while insights from the trauma model led me to view the ache in my chest as literal fragments of past pain (which in a way they were), meditation (buttressed by insights from neuroscience), showed me that this too could be said to be a construct. Is it the world that creates suffering, or the mind? It depends how you look at things. The two are not separate.

Catalysed by my breakthrough journey, the gap between my anxiety and the scripts my mind reeled about it got gradually wider, as sensation increasingly got decoupled from story. Internal phenomena that I'd once experienced as emotions could increasingly be seen as contentless patterns of activation, and often I would catch myself assuming I was having intrusive thoughts before realising that I was merely experiencing the old knot in my chest that used to be associated with them. The flashes grew softer, the booms grew quieter and the gaps between them grew longer and longer until the storm seemed to be passing over the horizon.

But are you ever *healed*? Past tense? It's a question that can be answered with another question: what do we mean by healed? If being healed means no longer being constantly tormented by your own psychology, then yes. If it means (and this is my favourite definition) the ability to be fully present for the most meaningful relationships in your life, then yes. If being healed means that the valence of your inner life is more positive and neutral than negative, then yes. If being healed means the privilege of not having every jot of energy sucked up by a preoccupation with your own misery, then yes.

But if being healed means living in reciprocal, non-transactional community, then no. If being healed is regularly feeling at one with nature, then no. If it means having a deep, all-body trust that your family and closest friends are as safe as they can be; that everyone within a stone's throw of where you live has secure housing and nutritious food; and that the natural world will still be healthy in half a century or less, then of course not. If this sounds earnest or parochial then so be it. We're so lost in irony in the West, we forget that for many people in traditional societies, the idea of an individual being healed in such a context would be perverse.

We all approach our individual healing journeys as individual units. We go to solo therapy. The question we're asking ourselves is always 'what can I get?', it is never 'what can I give?'. In wellness culture, we are encouraged to see ourselves, as Rob Burbea said, as 'centres of acquisition'[6]. We are always seeking to acquire answers, insights, remedies, solutions that solve *our* personal problems. And that's of course understandable if your problems are incapacitating you. We take it as a fact that talking about our mental health is the best thing for our mental health. What if it isn't? What if relentlessly focussing on our healing is part of why it's so hard to heal?

Before the pandemic, I had been volunteering at my local hospital and I loved it. After the service started again post-Covid, I meant to re-enrol but didn't. It was on my to do list for months. Some small, miserly, excuse-making part of me was able to deprioritise the task and eventually just not bother. What was the block in my heart that I couldn't get over? Why am I selfish? Why is it so hard to give? No psychotherapy ever showed much interest in the question of how to live an ethical life, but maybe this question is just as important as the one I was presented with: 'how do I get better?' Maybe the answer to the latter puzzle could at least in part have been found through an engagement with the former? Or maybe this is the benefit of hindsight talking and I'm forgetting how urgently unwell I was, and how, sometimes, you can barely open your eyes to look at the world, let alone philosophise about your contribution to it. I don't know. But again, I wonder if the psych industry has closed the door too firmly against the traditional religious values of reciprocity and duty that once offered communities a sense of purpose and selflessness that was naturally thera-peutic.

~

Psilocybin's power is its paradoxical ability to shatter indi-vidual self and work through it. Fearing that you are dying – a common experience on psilocybin and LSD – can be the viewfinder through which you discover how profoundly lucky you are to be alive. Mysteriously, my most healing threshold experience was the one that had nothing to do with me: a glowing orb entity announcing that I was crossing into a reality of human consciousness beyond thought. Seemingly, my defensive ego temporarily died. It was only through this 'death pathway'[7] as Malidoma Somé said, this reminder of the insignificance of my own story, that I was ironically able to see the significance of my personal injuries, receive the salve I needed ('Mommy's okay'), then give it all up.

Trauma culture encourages us to think about the causes of our suffering, and this can be fruitful. But it's easy to get stuck in trauma narratives, like the people in Plato's allegory who get stuck in the cave of their own psychology, under the illusion that their worldview is complete. Psychiatrist Dan Siegel invites us to ultimately relax the search for causality:

> Sometimes we need to get out of our own way, in order to not cause impediments to self-organisation . . . [which] needs no conductor, no programmer, no chairperson of the board to direct the show. There is no need to evoke a causal agent, one in charge, the director . . . It can be helpful to reflect on our longing for identifying causal relationships, and let them go.[8]

This points to why it's important not to direct the contents of your trips too much, and to go in with an openness to being surprised, since the power of psychedelics is their ability to challenge what we thought we understood. There was no way that I could've asked for the reassurance that I received in that last trip. I didn't know there was a part of me that thought Mom was dying. A part that was still waiting to find out if she was coming home. My adult-self knew for a fact that she hadn't been hospitalised for over a decade. I didn't know that a part of me didn't know that.

Here again, I find the prism image helpful. Healing itself is prismatic, a constant process of being surprised by a spectrum of colours, intricacies, and subversions I initially couldn't see. What if the healing prism was our go-to metaphor over the healing journey? Like metaphor itself, which opens out understanding by defining one thing in terms of another, healing is a process of complexification. An opposite action to the funnelling and simplification of the reducing valve which makes us rigid, closed and stuck in the first place.

In the months that followed my brief death of ego, I found that my past was unlocking without effort and everything was becoming smoother. The symptoms of what I would once have called body dysmorphic disorder improved, as I ceased to see my body as a series of disconnected parts to be scrutinised and started to see it as a whole. The double bind of my past selves' refusal to uproot and my present self's reluctance to abandon them became looser, as a sense of blending between all parts of me increased.

I could see now why my inner child had not wanted to budge from that house: she hadn't wanted to leave Mom alone. She'd been compelled to keep vigil there and had therefore been faced with an impossibility: to be wholly in the past and wholly in the present. In around 1611, my boy John Donne wrote one of the most beautiful poems about separation ever written, 'A Valediction: Forbidding Mourning'. When we're separated from someone we love, he says, we are never truly separated, the soul we share does not break or breach, it expands and spreads out, like a lump of gold beaten to a single atom thickness:

> Our two souls therefore, which are one,
>   Though I must go, endure not yet
> A breach, but an expansion,
>   Like gold to airy thinness beat.[9]

When I looked out over the ocean that one summer, feeling flat like the horizon, I wasn't just wondering how Mom was doing, I was in the room with her. The separation was real and not real at the same time. My OCD had projected that impossibility with constant simulations of the choices I could be making, the feelings I could be feeling, the identities I could be embracing. I'd found a psychological way of bridging the schism, living two lives at once, this life and the life not lived.

In the wake of my breakthrough journey, I no longer had to split my psyche across time and space now that I'd got the message: *Mommy's okay, Mommy's okay, Mommy's okay.* The words rained down their compassion on me for months following the trip, having become tethered to new bodily sensations of lightness and calm, as the mind–body system's astonishing predictive power laid down new associations and new constructed realities, reorganising, turning the mechanisms of misery into the mechanisms of joy.

Narrative structure is always modelling these mechanisms to us, whether we notice it or not. Stories show us that no matter how alone we feel, someone has trod this path before. When they make us laugh or move us to tears, stories show us that our unfolding is inseparable from everybody else's. Take the story of Dumbo.

In 2023, just before I submitted the final draft of this book, I watched the Disney film again for the first time in thirty years. I was curious to see it after so long because the little elephant had kept popping up as a motif in my writing, which had surprised me. I wasn't aware of having found the story particularly resonant as a child. Beyond the fact that

Dumbo eventually flew without the help of his 'magic' feather, I couldn't remember the ins and outs of the plot.

Dumbo and his mother live in cages in a travelling circus. Their nature and freedoms are curtailed. They have no choice but to do difficult, draining work. The clowns at the circus don't see the elephants' suffering. They think that elephants are made of rubber and are therefore incapable of feelings. Before Dumbo had arrived, his mother had already undergone great hardship. When, one day, she gets distressed and angry at yet more injustice, she is taken away and locked up alone in the madhouse. But she's not crazy, as Timothy Mouse comforts Dumbo, she's just broken-hearted.

But Dumbo is inconsolably sad. When he visits his mother one night, she cradles him in her trunk through the cage bars, but there's nothing he can do to help her. To make things worse, he has these big, stupid, floppy ears, which he hates, which embarrass him, which continue to sabotage him by tripping him up. One night, after accidentally ingesting a drug, Dumbo has a bizarre, altered state of consciousness, in turns playful and menacing, in which trickster pink elephants menace and entice him.

When Dumbo wakes up from the trip, there's been an astonishing change. With the help of Timothy Mouse who's always believed in him, Dumbo takes a leap of faith, casts off the feather he doesn't need, and discovers he can fly. Those big ears that he hated and that had caused him so much pain, are the very thing that, when embraced, become his wings. In the final beat of the story, mechanisms of misery become mechanisms of joy, as his marvellous flight buys him the liberation and safety of his mother.

And so, through a story written halfway across the world eight decades ago, I discovered what this book truly is at root: an enactment of the help I couldn't offer then. It's not a coincidence that we see ourselves reflected in timeless stories – they express our unconscious structures, and speak to parts of us that we don't know exist. But we must always be prepared to have the reflection disrupted.

Something else stuck from the moment I opened my eyes the morning after the psilocybin wore off, a crystal-clear message: *move on*. The trip had broken my heart wide open; the challenge now was for me to figure out how to live from that place of open-heartedness once the pyrotechnics faded, through mundane everyday life, through experiment and relationship and boring incremental change. The mushrooms were not going to do that for me. I had to step into my own agency.

On people's tendency to get hooked on tripping, Alan Watts famously said, 'When you get the message, hang up the phone. For psychedelic drugs are simply instruments, like microscopes, telescopes, and telephones. The biologist does not sit with eye permanently glued to the microscope; he goes away and works on what he has seen.'[10]

Storytellers know the importance of cutting the sentences and scenes they're most attached to, their *darlings*, since it's probably these that are interrupting the flow of the story. Much of this book has been a call for psychiatry to do the same: to take out the red pen and honestly appraise which hangovers from older drafts no longer work. That's very complicated, because on those darlings are hung prestige, careers, influencer profiles, and entire economies. We've hung our own capital on them too. We think that if we take on the identity of a diagnosed person or a traumatised person, then we will be accepted and understood. These lenses can be helpful, but they can also hold us back.

The mushrooms seemed to be saying: kill your darlings. Don't let the search for trauma become your identity. Keep shedding each new skin before it hardens. Infantilise yourself as much as you need to connect to your child-self but live like the resilient grown-up that you are. Resist meanings as much as you make them. Step away from the mirror. Don't get certain. Explore concepts if they're useful but always return with curiosity to the non-conceptual realm of the body, where the truth about what's happening is observable in every moment. Stop *doing the work* and start living. Stop the healing quest. Stop the journey. Stop grasping for the end of a story that you had all along. As I wrote in 2020 on a massive dose of MDMA: 'you don't have to search any more, you're already here.'

~

With some trepidation, I returned in 2022 to Bushey Fields, where my mother had repeatedly been taken when I was a child. I was visiting two of our family friends, a husband and wife, who had both been admitted at the same time. It hadn't changed. The same glaring strip lights, the same plastic chairs, the same plastic knives that snapped in hard butter, the same prison-like entry protocol.

As my dad and I walked through the lounge area, I looked at the table where we used to sit when we visited Mom, and was reminded of the last time I'd been here. It was in 2012 and Dad had brought a cutting for Mom from *The Times* by their favourite political cartoonist, depicting the speaker of the House of Commons headbutting his own reflection in a mirror. Mom had glanced at it, covered it with her hands and bit her lip. I'd looked at her questioningly and leaned in for an explanation. A fellow patient a few tables down had just been sedated for repeatedly headbutting staff.

I looked down at the comic cartoon of this flying headbutt, then across the room through the hushed politeness of visiting hours towards the patient who was sitting in the corner, drugged and smiling. It was such a tragic juxtaposition of images, and I was so tired and sad, that I burst into stifled laughter, which quickly turned into tears. Me, Mom, and Dad sat there, crying, laughing, at the awful absurdity and pain of this place and our predicament, taking in those giggles like air.

I've sometimes felt dragged down by a sense of negligence: of having, in my heart and in my previous memoir, neglected to honour the stories in my parents' and grandparents' generations by painting my struggles as an isolated disease, separate from, indifferent to, and unaffected by, everything they went through. I have felt angry at the way the mental health system treated my mother. At the way the education system treated my brother. At the government policies that decimated large swatches of the Midlands and put my dad out of work. I didn't know I was angry until, on psychedelics, the anger came scorching up from the centre of the earth and through me.

There's a fine therapeutic balance to be found between opening to anger and getting lost in its energy. Sometimes it's appropriate to let my child-self rage, to treat anger as a concrete and justified thing, and show how her story was shaped, beyond her control by external forces. Sometimes it's appropriate to deconstruct anger and see through it, to strip it of its power. Meditation and psychedelics can allow us to observe that the past, after all, does not exist anywhere but at the level of cognition and sensation in our own mind and body, where moment to moment we perpetuate it.

Through various altered states, I've been able to observe that a negative emotion is not a fixed thing, it is an always shifting profile of physical sensations: a twinge behind my ribs, a tightness in my jaw, a potentiality in my limbs. An abstraction, the constituent parts of which have no permanence; and that it's my reluctance to feel any given emotion that keeps it alive. For a long time, part of me wanted to keep my pain alive because, in a way, it anchored me to the people I love. To love deeply is to naturally feel distress when your family are wronged by forces stacked against them. But to receive love deeply, which is trickier, is to trust that those people, in their boundless love for you, would want nothing more than for you to be unburdened of pointless pain.

So much in our mental health conversation encourages us to analyse what's happened to us or what's wrong with us; to reduce ourselves to our upbringing or our brain chemistry. When we hit on something which rings true, we can be certain that we finally understand ourselves, and insist that others adopt that same understanding. Our credulity can then limit our openness to new perspectives, as mine did. Drip by drip, we form stories upon existing stories, until they solidify into stalagmites and keep us trapped in the cave, blocked off from the reality of who we really are. If you trust yourself enough and the universe enough, if you love yourself enough and you are loved enough, you can map your way out to a world of possibilities. Not by clinging to any one of your old stories, but by relaxing your grip and moving into the space and light between them.

Acknowledgements

I invited a small group of trusted readers to pull my manuscript apart. Their generous and thoughtful feedback notes were invaluable in making this book better. Huge thanks to Mohammed Ahmed, Folarin Sagaya, Alex Curmi, Tehseen Noorani, Joyce Blake, Jack Arbuthnott, Dad, Aaron Harvey and Emily Hayward Whitlock. Thank you to Ann Bissell at the Borough Press for believing in this almost unpitchable book from the start. And to Amy Perkins for so much expert guidance. Thank you to my agents and friends Crystal Mahey-Morgan and Jason Morgan for your passion and support. To the geeks and Romantics of the psychedelics underground, who've enriched my life no end; and to each interviewee for your time, wisdom and trust. Thank you to my family for once again giving me the freedom to tell a little of our story to the world. I love you.

Notes

1 Jack Kornfield, *After the Ecstasy, The Laundry: How the Heart Grows Wise on the Spiritual Path*, Sounds True, 2015

Intentions

1 Martha Newson et al., '"I Get High With a Little Help From My Friends" – How Raves Can Invoke Identity Fusion and Lasting Co-operation via Transformative Experiences', *Frontiers in Psychology* 12, 2021. https://www.frontiersin.org/articles/10.3389/fpsyg.2021.719596/full, accessed 2022

2 Shayne A. P. Dahl, 'Sleep Deprivation and the Vision Quest of Native North America', in Glaskin, K., Chenhall, R. (eds) *Sleep Around the World. Culture, Mind, and Society*, Palgrave Macmillan, pp.171–87, *Springer Link*, https://link.springer.com/chapter/10.1057/9781137315731_10, accessed 2023

3 Abraham H. Maslow, *Religions, Values and Peak Experiences*, Viking, 1970, https://www.atpweb.org/jtparchive/trps-02-70-02-083.pdf, accessed 2023

4 Malidoma Somé, *Of Water and Spirit*, New World Library, 2013

5 Ayon Maharaj, 'The challenge of the oceanic feeling: Romain Rolland's mystical critique of psychoanalysis and his call for a "new

science of the mind"', *History of European Ideas* 43,5, pp.474–93, https://philarchive.org/archive/MAHTCO-17, accessed 2022

6 Maximo Baquiran and Yasir Al Khalili, 'Lysergic Acid Diethylamide Toxicity', National Library of Medicine, https://www.ncbi.nlm.nih.gov/books/NBK553216, accessed 2023

7 Alan Watts, 'Q&A With God' [talk], https://www.organism.earth/library/document/q-and-a-with-god, 1971

8 Gregory Bateson, 'Consciousness & Psychopathology', YouTube, 5 August 2019, https://www.youtube.com/watch?v=IoHzywwSQUo&ab_channel=Insights, accessed 2022

9 Department for Culture, Media & Sport, 'Community Life Survey 2021/22: Wellbeing and loneliness', gov.uk, updated 3 May 2023, https://www.gov.uk/government/statistics/community-life-survey-202122/community-life-survey-202122-wellbeing-and-loneliness, accessed 2022

10 World Health Organization, 'Mental Health / Burden', World Health Organization, https://www.who.int/health-topics/mental-health#tab=tab_2, accessed 2022

11 Carl Baker, House of Commons Library, 'Suicide Statistics', UK Parliament, 2 December 2022, https://commonslibrary.parliament.uk/research-briefings/cbp-7749/, accessed 2023

12 Abraham H. Maslow, *The Psychology of Science: A Reconnaissance*, Harper & Row, 1966, p.15

13 National Institute for Health and Care Excellence (NICE), 'Common Mental Health Problems: identification and pathways to care' [CG123] NICE, 25 May 2011. https://www.nice.org.uk/guidance/cg123/ifp/chapter/common-mental-health-problems, accessed 2023

14 Michael E. Newman, 'Schizophrenia is a Disease, Not an Extreme of Normal Variation', *Johns Hopkins Medicine* 29 January 2020. https://www.hopkinsmedicine.org/news/newsroom/news-releases/schizophrenia-is-a-disease-not-an-extreme-of-normal-variation, accessed 2022

15 Therese O'Donoghue, 'A critical narrative analysis of psychiatrists' engagement with psychosis as a contentious area', *International Journal of Social Psychiatry* 66,7. 724–30. https://journals.sagepub.com/doi/full/10.1177/0020764020934516, accessed 2023

16 Hearing Voices Network, 'About Voices and Visions', *Hearing Voices Network*, https://www.hearing-voices.org/voices-visions/about, accessed 2023

17 Joseph Campbell, in Stanley Keleman and Joseph Campbell, *Myth and the Body: a colloquy with Joseph Campbell*, Center Press, 1999, p.7

18 Iain McGilchrist, *The Master and his Emissary: The Divided Brain and the Making of the Western World*, Audible Studios, 2020

Departure

1 Frank Tallis, *The Act of Living*, Hachette Audio UK, 2021

2 Jared R. Lindah et al., 'A phenomenology of meditation-induced light experiences: traditional Buddhist and neurobiological perspectives', *Frontiers in Psychology* 4, 2013, https://www.frontiersin.org/articles/10.3389/fpsyg.2013.00973/full, accessed 2023

3 David Veale and Alison Roberts, 'Obsessive-compulsive Disorder', *British Medical Journal* 34, 2014, https://www.bmj.com/content/348/bmj.g2183.full, accessed 2023

4 Alain de Botton, in The School of Life, *On Mental Illness*, 2022, p.163

Threshold

1 John O'Donohue, *The Inner Landscape*, Sounds True, 2015

2 Claire M. Gillan, 'Characterizing a psychiatric symptom dimension related to deficits in goal-directed control', *eLife* 5, 2016, National Library of Medicine, https://www.ncbi.nlm.nih.gov/pmc/articles/PMC4786435, accessed 2022

3 Dr Claire Gillan and Rose Cartwright, MQ Open Mind [podcast], 27 September 2017, https://mqopenmind.podbean.com/e/a-new-way-of-thinking-about-ocd

4 Arpit Parmar and Siddharth Sarkar, 'Neuroimaging Studies in Obsessive Compulsive Disorder: A Narrative Review', *Indian Journal of Psychological Medicine* 38(5), 2016, https://ncbi.nlm.nih.gov/pmc/articles/PMC5052949, accessed 2023

5 Boyle M. (2013), 'The persistence of medicalisation: Is the presentation of alternatives part of the problem?', Coles S., Keenan S., Diamond B. (Eds.), *Madness contested: Power and practice* (pp. 3-22), Ross-on-Wye, England: PCCS Books.

6 Adam Rogers, 'Star Neuroscientist Tom Insel Leaves the Google-Spawned Verily for . . . a Startup?', *WIRED*, 11 May 2017, https://www.wired.com/2017/05/star-neuroscientist-tom-insel-leaves-google-spawned-verily-startup/, accessed 2022

7 C. Pierce Salguero, '"This Fathom-Long Body": Bodily Materiality and Ascetic Ideology in Medieval Chinese Buddhist Scriptures', National Library of Medicine, https://pubmed.ncbi.nlm.nih.gov/29961714, accessed 2023

8 World Health Organization, 'Mental Disorders', WHO, 8 June 2022, https://www.who.int/news-room/fact-sheets/detail/mental-disorders, accessed 2022 and Global Burden of Disease, https://www.healthdata.org/research analysis/gbd#:~:text=The%20Global%20Burden%20of%20Disease,be%20improved%20and%20disparities%20eliminated, accessed 2023

Repeat beats

1 Henri Bergson, *Creative Evolution*, Routledge, 2022

2 John Donne, 'Death's Duel', https://www.online-literature.com/donne/3915, accessed 2023

3 John Donne, 'Meditation XVII, Devotions Upon Emergent Occasions', *The Norton Anthology Of English Literature*, W.W. Norton and Company, 1968, p.917

4 Ibid.
5 Shunryu Suzuki, quoted in 'Buddhism's Most Basic Teaching: Everything Changes', *The Dewdrop*, 19 April 2021, https://thedewdrop.org/2021/04/19/everything-changes-shunryu-suzuki, accessed 2022

Philospher's stones

1 Ajahn Chah, *Food for the Heart: The Collected Teachings of Ajahn Chah*, Audible Studios, 2016
2 James Hillman and Michael Ventura, *We've Had a Hundred Years of Psychotherapy and the World's Getting Worse*, HarperCollins, 1993, p.196
3 Michael Pollan, *How To Change Your Mind: What the New Science of Psychedelics Teaches Us About Consciousness, Dying, Addiction, Depression, and Transcendence*, Allen Lane, 2018
4 Emerson Dameron, 'Johns Hopkins studying effects of psilocybin on brains of long-term meditators', *Psymposa*, 22 November 2017, https://www.psymposia.com/magazine/johns-hopkins-studying-effects-of-psilocybin-on-brains-of-long-term-meditators, accessed 2021
5 Humphrey Osmond, 'A Review of the Clinical Effects of Psychotomimetic Agents', *Annals of the New York Academy of Sciences*, 66(3), 1957, pp. 418–434.
6 Aldous Huxley, *The Doors of Perception*, Vintage, 1954, p.11
7 David Nutt, 'Equasy – An overlooked addiction with implications for the current debate on drug harms', Sage Journals, https://journals.sagepub.com/doi/10.1177/0269881108099672, accessed 2023
8 David Nutt, Leslie A. King, and Lawrence D. Phillips, 'MCDA Comparison of Drug and Alcohol Harms in the UK', *Drug Science*, 1 November 2010, https://www.drugscience.org.uk/drug-harms-in-the-uk/, accessed 2023

Magic

1 David Whyte, 'Help', *Consolations: The Solace, Nourishment and Underlying Meaning of Everyday Words*, Canongate Books, 2019

2 Stanley Keleman, *Myth and the Body: a colloquy with Joseph Campbell*, Center Press, 1999, p.xiv

3 Bessel van der Kolk, *The Body Keeps the Score: Brain, Mind, and Body in the Healing of Trauma*, Penguin, 2014, p.97

4 Stephen King, *On Writing*, Hodder & Stoughton, 1967, p.143

Night sea journey

1 Carl Jung, *The Psychology of the Transference*, Princeton University Press, 1966

2 Carl Hart, *Drug Use For Grown Ups*, Penguin Audio, 2021

3 Sean Lawlor, 'Psychedelic Exceptionalism and Reframing Drug Narratives: An Interview with Dr. Carl Hart', *Psychedelics Today*, https://psychedelicstoday.com/2020/02/18/psychedelic-exceptionalism-and-reframing-drug-narratives-an-interview-with-dr-carl-hart, accessed 2023

4 Sylvia Plath, *The Bell Jar*, Faber & Faber, 2005, p. 2

5 James Hillman and Michael Ventura, *We've Had a Hundred Years of Psychotherapy and the World's Getting Worse*, HarperCollins, 1993, p.127

Subplot

1 John Berger in conversation with Susan Sontag, 'To Tell a Story', *Voices* [television programme], series 1, episode 7, Channel 4, 9 February 1983. YouTube, https://www.youtube.com/watch?v=MoHCR8nshe8&ab_channel=Everythinghasitsfirsttime, accessed 2022

2 Carl Jung, *The Psychology of the Transference*, Princeton University Press, 1966

3 Michael Pollan and Rose Cartwright, *The Libreria Podcast* [podcast], Second Home, 8 July 2019, https://share.transistor.fm/s/3069b85b

Connective tissue

1 Daniel Siegel, *IntraConnected: MWe (Me + We) as the Integration of Self, Identity, and Belonging*, Brilliance Audio, 2022

2 Kurt Vonnegut, Slaughterhouse 5, Vintage, 2000, p.142

3 Kurt Vonnegut, Slaughterhouse 5, Vintage, 2000, p.143

4 Oprah Winfrey, Dr Bruce Perry, *What Happened to You? Conversations on Trauma, Resilience, and Healing*, Bluebird, 2021

5 The Gottman Institute, 'The Research: The Still Face Experiment', https://www.gottman.com/blog/research-still-face-experiment, accessed 2023

6 Jason G. Goldman, 'Ed Tronick and the "Still Face Experiment"', *Scientific American*, 18 October 2010, https://blogs.scientificamerican.com/thoughtful-animal/ed-tronick-and-the-8220-still-face-experiment-8221, accessed 2022

7 Paul Conti, MD, *Trauma: The Invisible Epidemic: How Trauma Works and How We Can Heal from It*, Recorded Books, 2021

8 Nick Haslam, Jesse S.Y. Tse and Simon De Deyne, 'Concept Creep and Psychiatrization', *Frontiers in Sociology* 2021 6, https://www.ncbi.nlm.nih.gov/pmc/articles/PMC8716590/, accessed 2022

9 Johanna Bick and Charles A. Nelson, 'Early Adverse Experiences and the Developing Brain', *Neuropsychopharmacology* 41, 2016, *Nature*, https://www.nature.com/articles/npp2015252 accessed 2023

10 Frank Tallis, *The Act of Living: What the Great Psychologists Can Teach Us About Surviving Discontent in an Age of Anxiety*, Hachette Audio UK, 2021

11 Tehseen Noorani, interviewed by Rose Cartwright, 8 September 2023

12 Rose Cartwright, *Pure*, Unbound, 2015, p.13

13 David Whyte, 'Denial', *Consolations: The Solace, Nourishment and Underlying Meaning of Everyday Words*, Canongate Books, 2019

Matches

1 Hans Christian Andersen, *The Little Match Girl*, https://andersen. sdu.dk/vaerk/hersholt/TheLittleMatchGirl_e.html, The Hans Chistian Andersen Centre, accessed 2023

2 Nadav Liam Modlin, 'Clearing A Path for Treatment: The Importance of Facilitators and Therapists', Psych Symposium [conference], London, 6 July 2023

3 Ibid.

4 Timmy Davis interviewed by Rose Cartwright, 13 June 2023

5 Stephan Bodian, 'Elaborating on the direct approach', https://www. stephanbodian.org/blog/2021/10/9/elaborating-on-the-direct-approach#:~:text=Unlike%20thinking%2C%20direct%20sensation %20is,an%20imaginary%20past%20or%20future, accessed 2023

6 *Jurassic Park* [DVD], Director Stephen Spielberg, Universal Studios, 1993

7 George Lakoff and Mark Johnson, *Metaphors We Live By*, The University of Chicago Press, 1980, p.29

8 Rick Doblin, 'The future of psychedelic-assisted psychotherapy', TED, https://www.ted.com/talks/rick_doblin_the_future_of_ psychedelic_assisted_psychotherapy/transcript, accessed 2023

9 Alice Miller, *The Drama of the Gifted Child*, Basic Books, 2008, p.58

10 Gabor Maté, *In the Realm of Hungry Ghosts: Close Encounters with Addiction*, North Atlantic Books, 2010

11 The British Psychological Society and the Division of Clinical Psychology, *The Power Threat Meaning Framework*, January 2018, https://cms.bps.org.uk/sites/default/files/2022-07/PTM%20 Framework%20%28January%202018%29_0.pdf, accessed 2021

12 Tomi Ungerer, *Alumette*, L'Ecole des loisirs, 1997

The invisible hand

1 Rob Burbea, 'Heart Work', *Dharma Seed*, 8 August 2008, https:// dharmaseed.org/talks/9982, accessed 2022

2   Kasey Farris Windels, 'Proportional representation and regulatory focus : the case for cohorts among female creatives', University of Texas Libraries, 2008, https://repositories.lib.utexas.edu/handle/2152/17824, accessed 2022

3   William Shakespeare, Macbeth, Folger Shakespeare Library, https://www.folger.edu/explore/shakespeares-works/macbeth/read/3/2, accessed 2023

4   Emma Rothschild, 'Adam Smith and the Invisible Hand', *JSTOR*, 1994, https://www.jstor.org/stable/2117851, accessed 2022

5   Voices In Global Mental Health [conference], London, 11 November 2016

6   Martin Seager and Sue Baker, '1:4 and Stigma; Emotional Brain Training; Clio Barnard', *All In The Mind*, 11 November 2014, BBC Radio 4, https://www.bbc.co.uk/programmes/b04ntvvm, accessed 2019

7   Ibid.

8   Ibid.

9   Ashok Malla, Ridha Joober and Amparo Garcia, '"Mental illness is like any other medical illness": a critical examination of the statement and its impact on patient care and society', *Journal of Psychiatry & Neuroscience* 40 (3), May 2015, *National Library of Medicine*, https://www.ncbi.nlm.nih.gov/pmc/articles/PMC4409431/, accessed 2023

10 Sue Baker. Interview, Conducted by Rose Cartwright, 1 August 2023

11 Ethnicity facts and figures, 'Detentions Under the Mental Health Act', GOV.UK, 26 May 2023, https://www.ethnicity-facts-figures.service.gov.uk/health/mental-health/detentions-under-the-mental-health-act/latest, accessed 2023

12 Alexander Beiner, 'The Psychedelic Trojan Horse', Medium, 2021, https://medium.com/rebel-wisdom/the-psychedelic-trojan-horse-14c9704efd4, accessed 2023

As without, so within

1 John Berger, *Why Look at Animals?*, Penguin, 2009, p.52
2 Ibid., p.37
3 Ibid., p.52
4 Ibid., p.52

Healing in three acts

1 Joseph Campbell, in Stanley Keleman, *Myth and the Body: a colloquy with Joseph Campbell*, Center Press, 1999, p.3
2 Carl Rogers, *A Way of Being*, 1980, page number unknown
3 Joseph Campbell, *The Hero with a Thousand Faces*, New World Library, 2008, p.1
4 John Vervaeke, 'Plato and the Cave', *Awakening from the Meaning Crisis*, 15 February 2019, YouTube, https://www.youtube.com/playlist?list=PLND1JCRq8Vuh3f0P5qjrSdb5eC1ZfZwWJ, accessed 2022
5 Bootsy Collins, 'Bootsy's Basic Funk Formula', YouTube, https://www.youtube.com/watch?v=IHE6hZU72A4&ab_channel=Ediblspaceships', accessed 2013
6 *Dumbo* [DVD], Directors Samuel Armstrong, Norman Ferguson, Wilfred Jackson, Walt Disney, 1941
7 Carl Rogers, *A Way of Being*, 1980, page number unknown
8 Joseph Campbell, in Stanley Keleman, *Myth and the Body: a colloquy with Joseph Campbell*, Center Press, 1999, p.6
9 Joseph Campbell, in Stanley Keleman, *Myth and the Body: a colloquy with Joseph Campbell*, Center Press, 1999, p.xiii
10 Bessel van der Kolk, *The Body Keeps the Score*, Penguin, 2014, p.299
11 Ibid.
12 Ibid.
13 Kurt Vonnegut, 'On the Shapes of Stories', YouTube, https://www.youtube.com/watch?v=oP3c1h8v2ZQ&ab_channel=DavidComberg, accessed 2022

14 Joseph Campbell, in Stanley Keleman, *Myth and the Body: a colloquy with Joseph Campbell*, Center Press, 1999, p.xv

15 Jacqueline Anderson. Interview. Conducted by Rose Cartwright, 21 April 2023

16 Arnold Van Gennep, *The Rites of Passage*, University of Chicago Press, 1961

17 Malidoma Somé, *Of Water and Spirit*, New World Library, 2013

18 Ibid.

19 Malidoma Somé, *Of Water and Spirit*, New World Library, 2013

20 Allen Frances, 'Dungeons and Back Alleys: The Fate of the Mentally Ill in America', *Psychiatric Times* 36;10, 4 October 2019, https://www.psychiatrictimes.com/view/dungeons-and-back-alleys-fate-mentally-ill-america, accessed 2022

21 Future Care Capital, 'Europeans' use of antidepressants more than doubles in 20 years', *Future Care Capital*, 16 November 2022, https://futurecarecapital.org.uk/latest/europeans-use-of-antidepressants-doubles, accessed 2023

22 Campaign to End Loneliness, 'New analysis reveals people are more chronically lonely now than before Covid-19', *Campaign to End Loneliness*, 13 May 2022, https://www.campaigntoendloneliness.org/press-release/new-analysis-from-campaign-to-end-loneliness-reveals-people-are-more-chronically-lonely-now-than-before-covid-19, accessed 2023

23 NHS Digital, 'Mental Health of Children and Young People in England 2022 – wave 3 follow up to the 2017 survey', *NHS Digital*, 29 November 2022, https://digital.nhs.uk/data-and-information/publications/statistical/mental-health-of-children-and-young-people-in-england/2022-follow-up-to-the-2017-survey, accessed 2023

24 Malidoma Somé, *Of Water and Spirit*, New World Library, 2013

The bear hunt

1 Michael Rosen, *We're Going on a Bear Hunt*, Margaret K. McElderry Books, 2003

2 Dr Claire Gillan. Interview. Conducted by Rose Cartwright, 7 March 2022

3 George Bush, 'Project on the Decade of the Brain – Presidential Proclamation 6158', Library of Congress, 17 July 1990, https://www.loc.gov/loc/brain/proclaim.html, accessed 2022

4 Rose Cartwright, *Pure*, Audible Studios, 2020

5 Emily Bobrow, 'Psychiatrist Thomas Insel Looks for a Cure to America's Mental Health Crisis', *Wall Street Journal*, 11 February 2022, https://www.wsj.com/articles/psychiatrist-thomas-insel-looks-for-a-cure-to-americas-mental-health-crisis-11644600489, accessed 2022

6 Thomas Insel, 'The 'Nation's Psychiatrist' Takes Stock, With Frustration', *The New York Times*, https://www.nytimes.com/2022/02/22/us/thomas-insel-book.html, accessed 2023

7 Adam Rogers, 'Star Neuroscientist Tom Insel Leaves the Google-Spawned Verily for . . . a Startup?', *WIRED*, 11 May 2017, https://www.wired.com/2017/05/star-neuroscientist-tom-insel-leaves-google-spawned-verily-startup/, accessed 2022

8 Bessel van der Kolk, *The Body Keeps the Score: Brain, Mind, and Body in the Healing of Trauma*, Penguin, 2014, p.27

9 Ibid.

10 Sir Robin Murray, in response to Lucy Johnstone and Awais Aftab, 'Moving Beyond Psychiatric Diagnosis', *Psychiatric Times*, 14 August 2020, https://www.psychiatrictimes.com/view/moving-beyond-psychiatric-diagnosis-lucy-johnstone-psyd, accessed 2022

11 Joanna Moncrieff et al., 'The serotonin theory of depression: a systematic umbrella review of the evidence', *Molecular Psychiatry*, 2022, https://www.nature.com/articles/s41380-022-01661-0, accessed 2022

12 David Hellerstein, as quoted in E.J. Dickson, 'Who Is the Psychiatrist Behind the Antidepressant Study Taking Over Right-Wing Media?', *Rolling Stone*, 30 July 2022, https://www.rollingstone.com/culture/culture-news/ssri-right-wing-attack-joanna-moncrieff-1388067, accessed 2022

13 Joanna Moncrieff & Dr Ellie interview, *This Morning*, ITV, 21 July 2022

14 'The Antidepressant Story', Panorama, 19 June 2023, https://www. bbc.co.uk/iplayer/episode/m001n39z/panorama-the-antidepressant-story, accessed 2023

15 Professor Dainius Pūras, 'Right of everyone to the enjoyment of the highest attainable standard of physical and mental health', UN General Assembly, 2020, https://documents-dds-ny.un.org/doc/ UNDOC/GEN/G20/094/45/PDF/G2009445.pdf?OpenElement, accessed 2022

16 Awais Aftab, MD, 'Global Psychiatry's Crisis of Values: Dainius Pūras, MD', 2021, https://www.psychiatrictimes.com/view/global-psychiatry-crisis-values, accessed 2022

17 James Davies, 'Mental Health, Capitalism, and the Sedated of a Nation', *The Medicalisation of Distress* [conference], Confer, London, 4 March 2023, https://www.confer.uk.com/event/distress. html, accessed 2023

18 Kerryn Husk et al., 'Social prescribing: where is the evidence?', *British Journal of General Practice* 69 (678), January 2019 *National Library of Medicine*, https://www.ncbi.nlm.nih.gov/pmc/articles/ PMC6301369, accessed 2023

19 Ibid.

20 Professor Allen Frances referenced in Lucy Johnstone and Awais Aftab, 'Moving Beyond Psychiatric Diagnosis', *Psychiatric Times*, 14 August 2020, https://www.psychiatrictimes.com/view/moving-beyond-psychiatric-diagnosis-lucy-johnstone-psyd, accessed 2022

21 Miranda Fricker, 'Epistemic injustice resource page', University of Bristol, https://www.bristol.ac.uk/philosophy/research/epistemic-injustice-, accessed 2022

22 Dr Claire Gillan. Interview. Conducted by Rose Cartwright, 7 March 2022

23 Charles Foster, 'Charles Foster on *Being a Human: Adventures in Forty Thousand Years of Consciousness*', *The Michael Shermer Show* [podcast], Michael Shermer, 23 October 2021, https://www.skeptic.

com/michael-shermer-show/charles-foster-on-being-a-human-adventures-in-forty-thousand-years-of-consciousness, accessed 2021

24 Charles Foster, *Being A Human*, Profile Audio, 2021

25 Dr Claire Gillan. Interview. Conducted by Rose Cartwright, 7 March 2022

26 Sara Tai. Interview. Conducted by Rose Cartwright, 15 March 2022

27 Ibid.

Diagnostic dogma

1 Charles Foster, *Being A Human*, Profile Books, 2021, p.6

2 Allen Frances, interview. Conducted by Gary Greenberg, 'Inside the Battle to Define Mental Illness', *WIRED*, 27 December 2010, https://www.wired.com/2010/12/ff-dsmv, accessed 2022

3 Allen Frances, 'Saving Normal', *Psychology Today*, https://www.psychologytoday.com/gb/blog/saving-normal?, accessed 2022

4 Allen Frances, 'The Making of the DSM, An Insider's View', *Talking Therapy* [podcast], Allen Frances and Marvin Goldfried, May 2022, https://open.spotify.com/episode/2FzZck9DPOCzu9R6KPoB8f?si=C3H6xgy9QlGXVJSyx3A6Cw, accessed 2022

5 Andrew Jacobs, 'The Psychedelic Revolution Is Coming, Psychiatry May Never Be the Same', *New York Times*, 9 May 2021, https://www.nytimes.com/2021/05/09/health/psychedelics-mdma-psilocybin-molly-mental-health.html, accessed 2021

6 Andrew Scull, '"Scientific Nightmare": The Backstory of the "DSM"', *Los Angeles Review of Books*, 25 October 2021, https://lareviewofbooks.org/article/scientific-nightmare-the-backstory-of-the-dsm, accessed 2022

7 Multiple authors, *DSM-IV*, American Psychiatric Press Inc, 1994, p.xxxi

8 Ibid. p.xxx

9 Ibid. p.xxxi

10 Ibid. p.xxxiv

11 Allan V. Horrowitz, *DSM: A History of Psychiatry's Bible*, Tantor Audio, 2021

12 Hearing Voices Network, 'Basic Information about Voices and Visions', https://www.hearing-voices.org/voices-visions, accessed 2023

13 Lisa Feldman Barrett, How Emotions Are Made (Cinematic Lecture), 2020, https://www.youtube.com/watch?v=0rbyC5m557I&ab_channel=Flow, accessed 2023

14 Gregory Bateson, 'Consciousness & Psychopathology', YouTube, 5 August 2019, https://www.youtube.com/watch?v=IoHzyw-wSQUo&ab_channel=Insights, accessed 2022

15 Multiple authors, *DSM-IV*, American Psychiatric Press Inc, 1994, p.715

16 Ibid.

17 Alan Watts, The Tao of Philosophy, 1965, https://alanwatts.org/transcripts/the-tao-of-philosophy-5, accessed 2021

18 Marta Paterlini, 'There shall be order. The legacy of Linnaeus in the age of molecular biology', *EMBO Reports* 8(9), September 2007, on *National Library of Medicine*, https://www.ncbi.nlm.nih.gov/pmc/articles/PMC1973966, accessed 2023

19 Robin Carhart-Harris et al., 'Canalization and plasticity in psychopathology', *Neuropharmacology* 226, 15 March 2023, on *ScienceDirect*, https://www.sciencedirect.com/science/article/pii/S0028390822004579?via%3Dihub, accessed 2023

20 Robin Carhart-Harris et al., 'Canalization and plasticity in psychopathology', *Neuropharmacology* 226, 15 March 2023, on *ScienceDirect*, https://www.sciencedirect.com/science/article/pii/S0028390822004579?via%3Dihub, accessed 2023

21 Mason Schreck, 'Stanislav and Christina Grof: Cartographers of the Psyche', https://maps.org/news-letters/v21n3/v21n3-26_29.pdf, accessed 2023

22 Dr Sara Tai. Interview. Conducted by Rose Cartwright, 15 March 2022

23 Alex Curmi. Interview. Conducted by Rose Cartwright, 27 September 2022

24 Joyce Blake. Interview. Conducted by Rose Cartwright, 15 October 2023

25 Gabor Maté and Daniel Maté, *The Myth of Normal: Trauma, Illness & Healing in a Toxic Culture*, Vermilion, 2022

26 W. Thomas Boyce and Bruce J Ellis, 'Biological sensitivity to context: I. An evolutionary-developmental theory of the origins and functions of stress reactivity', *Development and Psychopathology* 17 (2), 2005, *National Library of Medicine*, https://pubmed.ncbi.nlm.nih.gov/16761546, accessed 2023

27 Euan Ward, 'After Gutting Youth Services, Can the U.K. Still Cut Youth Crime?', *New York Times*, 4 February 2023, https://www.nytimes.com/2023/02/04/world/europe/london-austerity-youth-violence.html, accessed 2023

28 Gabor Maté. Interview. Conducted by Rose Cartwright, 28 March 2023

Nonlinearity

1 Arnold Van Gennep, *The Rites of Passage*, University of Chicago Press, 1961

2 Annie Wright, 'What Is the Window of Tolerance, and Why Is It So Important?', 2022, https://www.psychologytoday.com/gb/blog/making-the-whole-beautiful/202205/what-is-the-window-tolerance-and-why-is-it-so-important, accessed 2023

3 Deb Dana, 'Understanding the Polyvagal Ladder', 2021, https://traumatherapistnetwork.com/understanding-the-polyvagal-ladder-a-brief-overview, accessed:2023

4 Kirby Reutter, 'Trauma stabilization through polyvagal theory and DBT', *Counselling Today*, 2021, https://ct.counseling.org/2021/09/trauma-stabilization-through-polyvagal-theory-and-dbt, accessed 2022

5 Cornelia Elbrecht, 'Pendulation as a Core Trauma Healing Model', 2022, https://www.sensorimotorarttherapy.com/blog/pendulation-as-a-core-trauma-healing-model, accessed 2023

6 R. D. Laing, *Knots*, Vintage Books, 1972, p.20

7 Donald Winnicott, 'Communicating and not communicating, leading to the studies of certain opposites – BPAS (not final version), 15 May 1963', in Robert Adès (ed.), *The Collected Works of D. W. Winnicott: Volume 12, Appendices and Bibliographies*, Oxford Academic online edn, 2016. https://academic.oup.com/book/12894/chapter/329240413, accessed 2023

8 Adele M. Hayes et al., 'Change is Not Always Linear: The Study of Nonlinear and Discontinuous Patterns of Change in Psychotherapy', National Library of Medicine, https://www.ncbi.nlm.nih.gov/pmc/articles/PMC3163164, accessed 2023

9 Dictionary of Psychology, 'Holding environment, American Psychological Association, https://dictionary.apa.org/holding-environment, accessed 2023

10 Dorothy E. Stubbe, 'The Therapeutic Alliance: The Fundamental Element of Psychotherapy', *Focus* 16 (4), at National Library of Medicine, https://www.ncbi.nlm.nih.gov/pmc/articles/PMC6493237, accessed 2023; American Psychological Association, 'Optimizing Therapy: What the evidence shows', *Monitor on Psychology* 50; 10, November 2019, https://www.apa.org/monitor/2019/11/ce-corner-sidebar, accessed 2023; Michael Lambert and Dean E. Barley, 'Research Summary of the Therapeutic Relationship and Psychotherapy Outcome', *Psychotherapy Theory Research Practice Training* 38(4), January 2001, https://www.researchgate.net/publication/232477357_Research_Summary_of_the_Therapeutic_Relationship_and_Psychotherapy_Outcome, accessed 2023

11 R. D. Laing, Practice and Theory – The Present Situation', *Psychotherapy and Psychosomatics, vol. 13*, 1965, *JSTOR*, http://www.jstor.org/stable/45111912, accessed 2023

12 Johns Hopkins Medicine, 'Hopkins scientists show hallucinogen in mushrooms creates universal "mystical" experience', *Eureka Alert*, 11 July 2006, https://www.eurekalert.org/news-releases/705464, accessed 2022

Back story

1 Joan Halifax, *The Fruitful Darkness: A Journey Through Buddhist Practice and Tribal Wisdom*, Audible Studios, 2015 https://www.audible.co.uk/pd/The-Fruitful-Darkness-Audiobook/B00X6GCME2

2 Joseph Rowntree Foundation, *UK Poverty 2022: The essential guide to understanding poverty in the UK*, 18 January 2022, https://www.jrf.org.uk/report/uk-poverty-2022, accessed 2022

3 Samaritans, *Dying from inequality: Socioeconomic disadvantage and suicidal behaviour, Summary Report* 2017, p.6, https://media.samaritans.org/documents/Samaritans_Dying_from_inequality_report_-_summary.pdf, accessed 2023

4 Ibid. p.4

5 NHS Digital, 'Mental Health of Children and Young People in England', 2020, https://files.digital.nhs.uk/AF/AECD6B/mhcyp_2020_rep_v2.pdf, accessed 2023

6 Institute of Health Equity, 'Health Equity in England, The Marmot Review 10 Years On', https://www.instituteofhealthequity.org/resources-reports/marmot-review-10-years-on/the-marmot-review-10-years-on-full-report.pdf, accessed 2023

7 Mental Health Foundation, 'People with learning disabilities: statistics', https://www.mentalhealth.org.uk/explore-mental-health/statistics/people-learning-disabilities-statistics, accessed 2023

8 Sandy E. James et al., *The Report of the 2015 U.S. Transgender Survey*, National Center For Transgender Equality, 2015, p.5, https://transequality.org/sites/default/files/docs/usts/USTS-Full-Report-Dec17.pdf, accessed 2023

9 Google Books Ngram Viewer, 'nervous breakdown', https://books.google.com/ngrams/graph?content=nervous+breakdown&year_start=1800&year_end=2019&corpus=en-2019&smoothing=3, accessed 2022

10 Jenny Useem, 'Bring Back the Nervous Breakdown', *The Atlantic*,

2021, https://www.theatlantic.com/magazine/archive/2021/03/bring-back-the-nervous-breakdown/617788, accessed 2023

11 Roy Richard Grinker, '*Roy Richard Grinker – Nobody's Normal: How Culture Created the Stigma of Mental Illness*', *The Michael Shermer Show* [podcast], Michael Shermer, 2 March 2021, https://www.skeptic.com/michael-shermer-show/roy-richard-grinker-nobodys-normal-how-culture-created-stigma-of-mental-illness, accessed 2022

12 Gareth Knott. Interview. Conducted by Rose Cartwright, 31 October 2022

13 Lambeth Together, *Lambeth Food Poverty and Insecurity Action Plan, 2021–2024*, Lambeth Council, February 2021, p.5, https://www.lambeth.gov.uk/sites/default/files/2021-01/Lambeth%20Food%20Poverty%20and%20Insecuity%20action%20plan%20final%20draft.pdf, accessed 2022

14 Gareth Knott. Interview. Conducted by Rose Cartwright, 31 October 2022

15 Interview. Conducted by Rose Cartwright, 11 July 2023

16 Joan Halifax, *The Fruitful Darkness: A Journey Through Buddhist Practice and Tribal Wisdom*, Audible Studios, 2015 https://www.audible.co.uk/pd/The-Fruitful-Darkness-Audiobook/B00X6GCME2

17 Good Things Foundation, '1.9 million are isolated by COVID-19 and are not online: we need to include them, now!', https://www.goodthingsfoundation.org/what-we-do/news/1-9-million-are-isolated-by-covid-19-and-are-not-online-we-need-to-include-them-now, accessed 2023

18 Dr Peter Kinderman. Interview. Conducted by Rose Cartwright, 18 February 2022

19 Marcus Aurelius Antoninus, *The Meditations of the Emperor Marcus Aurelius Antoninus*, Google Books, 2018, https://google.com.au/books/edition/The_Meditations_of_the_Emperor_Marcus_Au/gi1stAEACAAJ?hl=en, accessed 2023

20 William Shakespeare, *Hamlet*, Penguin, 2015, Act II. Scene II, 268-274

21 Daniel David, Ioana Cristea and Stefan G. Hofmann, 'Why Cognitive Behavioral Therapy Is the Current Gold Standard of Psychotherapy', *Frontiers in Psychiatry* 29, January 2018, at National Library of Medicine, https://www.ncbi.nlm.nih.gov/pmc/articles/PMC5797481, accessed 2023

22 Dr Peter Kinderman. Interview. Conducted by Rose Cartwright, 18 February 2022

23 Dr James Davies (@JDaviesPhD) 'The psychological virtues of the neoliberal era . . .', Twitter, 20 February 2023, https://twitter.com/jdaviesphd/status/1627573769534316544?s=46&t=xO9je8dd_02pnppy28Dosg, accessed 2023

24 Dr Peter Kinderman. Interview. Conducted by Rose Cartwright, 18 February 2022

25 Gareth Knott. Interview. Conducted by Rose Cartwright, 31 October 2022

26 Allen Frances, 'Don't Blame the Patient', *Talking Therapy* [podcast], Allen Frances and Marvin Goldfried, 3 April 2023, https://www.youtube.com/watch?v=A-FdXpqnwCI&ab_channel=TalkingTherapy, accessed 2023

27 Dr Peter Kinderman. Interview. Conducted by Rose Cartwright, 18 February 2022

28 Robert Waldinger, 'The Long Game: A Conversation with Robert Waldinger', *Making Sense* [podcast], Sam Harris, 11 January 2023, https://www.samharris.org/podcasts/making-sense-episodes/308-the-long-game, accessed 2023

29 James Davies, 'Mental Health, Capitalism, and the Sedated of a Nation', The Medicalisation of Distress [conference], London, 4 March 2023, https://www.confer.uk.com/event/distress.html, accessed 2023

30 Derek Summerfield, 'The Impact of War and Atrocity on Civilian Populations: Basic Principles for NGO Interventions and a Critique of Psychosocial Trauma Projects', Relief and Rehabilitation Network, April 1996, p.15, https://odihpn.org/wp-content/uploads/1996/04/networkpaper014.pdf, accessed 2022

31 Adam Aronovich, 'How Western medicine and indigenous traditions differ in their approach to mental health and healing' [podcast], October 2020, https://www.plantmedicine.org/podcast/traditions-adam-aronovich, accessed 2023

32 John Vervaeke, 'Awakening from the Meaning Crisis – Higher States of Consciousness, Part 2' [podcast], https://www.meaningcrisis.co/ep-12-awakening-from-the-meaning-crisis-higher-states-of-consciousness-part-2-2, accessed 2022

33 Ibid.

34 Henry Shukman on Tim Ferriss, 'Henry Shukman – Zen, Tools for Awakening, Ayahuasca vs. Meditation, Intro to Koans, and Using Wounds as the Doorway', *The Tim Ferriss Show* [podcast], 8 September 2021, https://tim.blog/2021/09/08/henry-shukman, accessed 2023

I am because I party

1 Gregory Bateson, '*Pathologies of Epistemology*', *Steps to an Ecology of Mind*, University of Chicago Press, 1972, p.493

2 World Health Organization, Mental Health Atlas, https://www.who.int/publications/i/item/9789241514019, accessed 2023

3 Sacred Design Lab, *Design for the Human Soul*, October 2019, https://sacred.design/wp-content/uploads/2019/10/SDL_Design_TRACT_Digital_101119.pdf, accessed 2023

4 YoungMinds, 'Mental Health Statistics', https://www.youngminds.org.uk/about-us/media-centre/mental-health-statistics, accessed 2023

5 Nandita Chaudhary in Leberecht Funk et al., 'Feeding, Bonding, and the Formation of Social Relationships. Ethnographic Challenges to Attachment Theory and Early Childhood Interventions', *Elements in Psychology and Culture*, 21 July 2023, https://www.researchgate.net/publication/372497386_Feeding_Bonding_and_the_Formation_of_Social_Relationships_Ethnographic_Challenges_to_Attachment_Theory_and_Early_Childhood_Interventions, accessed 2023

6 Scott R. Huston, 'The Rave: Spiritual Healing in Modern Western Subcultures', *Anthropological Quarterly*, 73;1, January 2000, on *JSTOR*, https://www.jstor.org/stable/3317473, accessed 2023

7 The Streets, 'Weak Become Heroes', *Original Pirate Material*, 2002

8 Daniel J Siegel MD, IntraConnected, MWe (Me + We) as the Integration of Self, Identity, and Belonging, Brilliance Audio, 2022

9 James Hillman and Michael Ventura, We've Had a Hundred Years of Psychotherapy and the World's Getting Worse, HarperCollins, 1993, p.40

10 Gregory Bateson, 'Pathologies of Epistemology', *Steps to an Ecology of Mind*, University of Chicago Press, 1972, p.492

11 Ibid. p.491

Kill your darlings

1 John Yorke, *Into the Woods: How Stories Work and Why We Tell Them*, Penguin, 2014, p.72

2 Loch Kelly, 'No Problem to Solve', https://lochkelly.org/faq/watch, accessed 2023

3 Jerome Bruner, 'Life as Narrative', *Social Research* 54;1, 1987, *JSTOR*, https://www.jstor.org/stable/40970444, accessed 2023

4 Rob Burbea, 'Heart Work' [talk], Dharma Seed, 8 August 2008, https://dharmaseed.org/talks/9982, accessed 2022

5 Lisa Feldman Barrett, 'Lisa Feldman Barrett: Surprising Truths about the Human Brain', *The Psychology Podcast* [podcast], Scott Barry Kaufman, 25 November 2021, https://scottbarrykaufman.com/podcast/lisa-feldman-barrett-surprising-truths-about-the-human-brain, accessed 2022

6 Rob Burbea, 'Heart Work' [talk], *Dharma Seed*, 8 August 2008, https://dharmaseed.org/talks/9982, accessed 2022

7 Malidoma Somé, *Of Water and Spirit*, New World Library, 2013

8 Dan Siegel, MD, *Mind: A Journey to the Heart of Being Human*, Brilliance Audio, 2016

9 John Donne, 'A Valediction: Forbidding Mourning', https://www. poetryfoundation.org/poems/44131/a-valediction-forbidding-mourning, accessed 2023

10 Alan Watts, *The Joyous Cosmology: Adventures in the Chemistry of Consciousness*, New World Library, 2013.

Credits